DARK INTRUSIONS

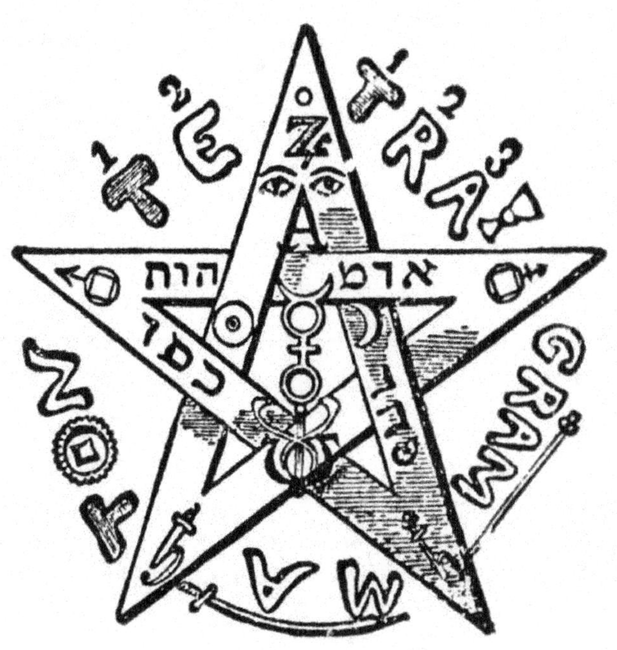

DARK INTRUSIONS

An Investigation into the Paranormal Nature of Sleep Paralysis Experiences

By Louis Proud

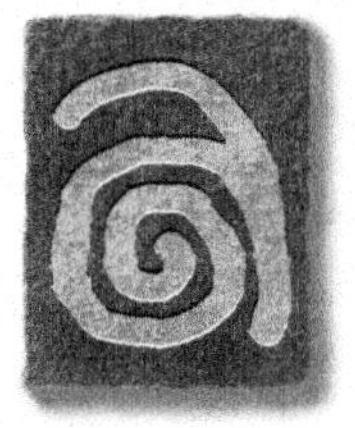

Anomalist Books
San Antonio * New York

An Original Publication of Anomalist Books

DARK INTRUSIONS

ISBN: 1933665440

Some material in this book first appeared in magazines. Permission has been granted to use this material. Portions of Chapter 5 and Chapter 6 were published in *Fate* magazine: Proud, Louis, "Poltergeists," *Fate*, January, 2008; Proud, Louis, "The Enfield Poltergeist Revisited," *Fate*, October, 2007. Portions of Chapter 1, Chapter 2, Chapter 5, Chapter 7, Chapter 8, Chapter 9, and Chapter 15 were published in *New Dawn* magazine: Proud, Louis, "Mind Parasites & the World of Invisible Spirits," *New Dawn*, Special Issue No. 3, Winter, 2007; Proud, Louis, "Allan Kardec and the Way of the Spirit," *New Dawn*, Special Issue No. 5, Winter 2008; Proud, Louis, "Haunted by Hungry Ghosts: The Joe Fisher Story," *New Dawn*, Special Issue No. 5, Winter, 2008; Proud, Louis, "Forces of the Unconscious Mind: Exploring the Work of Stan Gooch," *New Dawn* No. 105, Nov-Dec, 2007; Proud, Louis, "Chico Xavier: The Pope of Spiritism," *New Dawn,* Special Issue No. 6, Summer 2008/2009; Proud, Louis, "Aliens, Predictions & the Secret School: Decoding the Work of Whitley Strieber," *New Dawn*, Special Issue No. 4, Spring, 2008.

Permission has been granted by J. Allan Cheyne to quote from the University of Waterloo's Sleep Paralysis website.

Cover art by Robin Ray, courtesy of the Mary Evans Picture Library
Cover design by Crystal Hollis

Book design by Seale Studios

For information, go to anomalistbooks.com, or write to:
Anomalist Books, 5150 Broadway #108, San Antonio, TX 78209

Table of Contents

To the cruel, starved, and nameless ones who exist, "not in the spaces we know, but between them," and who, forever seeking warmth, forever seeking pleasure, forever seeking form, are drawn to the living like moths to a flame, drinking of our energy but gaining little nourishment. Long have you dwelt in darkness, friends. May you quit the night and seek the day. May you know something of happiness.

Foreword

By David J. Hufford, Ph.D.

Sleep paralysis is an episode of inability to move just before falling asleep or on awakening. It is usually brief. The paralysis is caused by the brain mechanism that paralyzes us during dreaming sleep (often called rapid eye movement sleep, or REM, in the sleep literature). This prevents dreamers from moving their physical body during dream movement, thereby preventing constant awakenings. This brief description sounds simple, but sleep paralysis itself has turned out to be very complex indeed!

When I began studying sleep paralysis in 1970 it was practically unknown outside of scientific sleep research and was thought to be quite rare, considered a symptom of the sleep disorder called narcolepsy. It was known that the experience was very frightening, and that sometimes people said that they had "seen things" during sleep paralysis. I encountered sleep paralysis in Newfoundland, Canada, while I was studying local folk beliefs as part of my doctoral dissertation. But I did not know, at first, that it was sleep paralysis that I had run into.

In Newfoundland they called it "the Old Hag." They described the paralysis, and they said that the helpless victim was then approached by an evil, malevolent entity. Some thought it was caused by witchcraft, others by ghosts. All agreed that it was terrifying and that it should be combated with traditional spiritual protections or charms. My research showed that in Newfoundland it was common for people to have this awful experience; around 20 percent of those in my surveys said it had happened to them. That was far too common for what I had read of sleep paralysis, and the Newfoundlanders reporting this attack had none of the symptoms of narcolepsy. But apart from the "Hag," the features of these attacks seemed indistinguishable from what the sleep research literature called sleep paralysis. Could this be a peculiarity of Newfoundland culture? Could sleep paralysis be given this bizarre "folk" content by local cultural tradition, and could that tradition somehow create a setting in which you needn't be narcoleptic to have the attack?

In graduate school I had learned the conventional view of alleged anomalous experiences that predicted such a process. In this view, which I call the Cultural Source Hypothesis, accounts of anomalous experience are produced by cultural models influencing the processes of story-telling, interpretation, and perception. From rumor to optical illusions to outright hallucinations, belief in the supernatural is said to produce experiences that appear to support those beliefs in a neatly circular fashion. I might have considered that possibility except for one thing: I had experienced the entire terrifying attack in Pennsylvania in 1963, as a college student, without ever having heard of "the Old Hag" or any such thing.

I had been awakened in my dark off-campus room by the sound of my door opening, and then footsteps approaching my bed. I tried to turn on my bedside light, but I found that I couldn't move. I felt the bed go down as if someone was climbing on it, and then I felt someone kneel on my chest. I felt I was being strangled and thought I would die. I struggled, not only against the physical threat, but also against a sense of revulsion at the thing on top of me. I had an overwhelming sense of evil from whatever was attacking me. Suddenly I broke through the paralysis, leaped out of bed, turned on the light – and found no one there. I was sure that I had been awake, and I was deeply puzzled. I did not discuss this, for the obvious reasons, until I crossed paths with that attacker again in Newfoundland. My own experience would not allow me to address this "folk belief" in the conventional way.

Over the following years, almost forty years now, I was able to show that the complex pattern of sleep paralysis, including the evil presence, the common shuffling footsteps, and a host of other details, does not arise from culture. Rather, in cultures around the world, traditions of spiritual assault arise from this experience. In Newfoundland they say that bad people who know how can "hag" you (*hag* is an old English term for witch). The person who is paralyzed is ridden by a hag – they are "hag rid," the origin of the term haggard – and one who has the experience repeatedly does rapidly become haggard! It is the hag on you that causes the pressure, sometimes a crushing sensation at the chest. In older English they called it the Mare, from the Anglo-Saxon root *merran*, "to crush." And eventually, the nightmare, the crusher who comes in the night. These very different terms – and the *da chor*, *dab coj*, *poj ntxoog*, or *dab tsog* in southeast Asia; the sitting ghost or *bei Guai chaak* (being pressed by a ghost) in China; in Japan the *kanashibari* ("metal bound" a Ninja practice comparable to the English term "spell bound"); the *Mara* of Sweden, and many more from around the world and throughout history – refer to the same event as the modern term sleep paralysis. But those traditions include a great deal more information – and conjecture – than does "sleep paralysis." The inadequacy of the conventional understandings of sleep paralysis, and the broad range cultural interpretations of it as a paranormal event around the world, are laid out and explored in my book, *The Terror That Comes in the Night.*

The experience itself is unimaginable to those who have not had it or heard of it from others, so clearly it is not a product of the imagination. But, then, what is it? The one thing certain is that it is still a mystery. There is no simple, conventional explanation. There are those who experience only paralysis, and they are the fortunate ones. But the great majority, more than three quarters of all who have the experience, encounter the evil presence. There are also those for whom the paralysis lasts more than a few seconds or a minute or two. Sometimes this turns into an out-of-body experience. In fact, shamans in some cultures cultivate sleep paralysis, overcoming their fear and the intimidation of the presence, as a method for leaving their bodies. In different cultures some of the specific details vary, as in whether the presence is a witch, a ghost, a demon, or an alien, but one thing does not vary. Most sleep paralysis experiences are replete with what appear to be paranormal details. The more one compares these episodes across subjects, the more paranormal they seem.

Louis Proud offers us a rare opportunity in *Dark Intrusions.* This insider's account of his own sleep paralysis experiences, in detail, is of great value. Then for that insider to knowledgeably place the experience in the broad paranormal context is unique. It provides a badly needed view of the cultural/interpretive framework that this experience naturally suggests. Louis Proud has been bold and thoughtful in providing this. Whether one accepts each of his conclusions or not, his book gives us an opportunity to see in detail the ways that sleep paralysis suggests connections to a wide variety of other anomalous phenomena.

Foreword
By Colin Wilson

Still in his twenties, Louis Proud has demonstrated with this book that he is one of the most acute commentators on the paranormal to appear in recent years. His starting point is the condition called sleep paralysis – shortened to SP – when someone wakes in the middle of the night and finds himself unable to move; a state that may last seconds or minutes.

When I mentioned it to my wife this morning, she said: "But surely that's purely a physical condition?" The answer is that it may be, but often is not.

Many "psychics" experience it as a prelude to an OBE, an out of the body experience. For example, Robert Monroe, founder of the Monroe Institute in Virginia, began to have them it in the late 1960s, when he was conducting personal experiments in "sleep learning." He began to experience what he called "vibrations" on the point of sleep. One day his hand, which was touching the floor, seemed to go through the carpet so he could feel the floor space below. And soon Monroe was having full-fledged OBEs. Obviously, the "vibrations" were a kind of disconnection from his senses, as if his "spirit" was separating from his physical body. Or – using a more down-to-earth analogy – a car had slipped out of gear and into ""neutral."

Louis Proud began to have similar experiences when he was 17. He says it is as if there is a malevolent presence nearby, sometimes as if something is squatting on the chest to prevent the sleeper from moving. Hallucinations, both visual and auditory, may also be experienced. Like my friend Stan Gooch, author of *Total Man,* Louis Proud has even had sexual encounters when in the SP state.

That certainly sounds as far from "normal" experience as one can get. Yet it is important to emphasize that many such experiences have a basis in normality. What makes Louis Proud's book so interesting is that he is obviously the kind of person who often has experiences that are beyond the normal. Yet his book is not a collection of weird oddities, but an exploration of the world that lies behind our eyes, yours as well as mine.

It seems clear to me that Louis Proud has been intrigued by his own paranormal experiences and is therefore more "open" to a remarkable range of them. So what he has done here is to gather together many strange experiences, like the Enfield poltergeist, Whitley Strieber's "contact" experiences, Stan Gooch's hypnogogic visions, Trevor Constable's UFO-related discarnates, Joe Fisher's mendacious and deceitful ghosts, Van Dusen's auditory hallucinations, and Dion Fortune's alarming contacts with an ill-disposed "witch," to make a book that grips the reader from beginning to end.

It seems to me immensely sad that the world should be polarized into hard-line skeptics – like "The Amazing Randi" – and people like myself who are perfectly willing to consider the paranormal as a reasonable possibility. Which is why, as I read Louis Proud's book, I began to feel a rising excitement, and the feeling: "This man is so obviously sincere that a reader would need to be pretty prejudiced to dismiss it all as self-delusion."

It gives me immense pleasure to be allowed to introduce a writer who will, I suspect, become widely admired for his enviable brilliance and clarity.

Introduction

When I was seventeen years old something changed within my mind; a shift of awareness occurred, and I became receptive to the presence of invisible beings – and I still am. Call them spirits if you like. Whenever I hear, feel, see, and sense these beings, I am always in an altered state of consciousness. Never am I fully awake. I do not have, and have never had, any kind of mental illness, nor am I on medication for any reason whatsoever; nor do I take recreational drugs.

The condition I suffer from is called sleep paralysis (SP), and it's not all that uncommon. About 25-to-40 percent of the population will undergo an SP episode at least once in the course of their life. The experience may be so minor, or may have occurred so many years ago, that it's now entirely forgotten, or remains but a dim memory. For some of us, however, these experiences occur frequently and cannot be forgotten. They have had, and continue to have, a profound impact on our spirituality.

So what is SP, and how is it associated with things that go bump in the night?

Explained simply, SP is a condition whereby a person experiences temporary paralysis of the body shortly after waking up (known as hypnopompic paralysis), and, less commonly, shortly after falling asleep (known as hypnagogic paralysis). Although their minds are reasonably awake and alert, they find themselves unable to move their bodies – sometimes for as long as a few minutes, though usually just for a few seconds.

The condition is closely related to the normal paralysis that occurs during REM (rapid eye movement) sleep – called muscle atonia – in which the body is paralyzed to inhibit a person from enacting dream activity, such as running while dreaming about running; this prevents us from causing ourselves physical harm. Some scientists and physicians believe it's a normal part of the sleep cycle. Generally, when SP occurs, the brain has awakened from an REM state, yet bodily paralysis is still taking place. In some instances, the sufferer may experience hypnopompic or hypnagogic hallucinations, which can be auditory, tactile, or visual in nature.

So there you have it – a neat and succinct explanation of SP. If you were to look up the subject in an encyclopedia or textbook, you would probably come across an explanation much like the one above. To this day, the phenomenon, particularly its spiritual side, remains little understood.

Any "expert" in these matters will smugly tell you that there is nothing more to SP than some temporary abnormal brain activity; that the hallucinations of SP sufferers are simply a product of the imagination. By holding such a view, however, one is almost denying the very existence of the phenomenon. My use of the term "hallucination" is only for simplicity's sake. I do not consider these experiences, for the most part, to be hallucinations.

During an SP attack, a person often feels that there is a malevolent presence nearby – sometimes perceived as a demon or evil spirit – and that this being is holding you down by resting on your chest, preventing you from moving or fully waking up. The sensation is very uncomfortable and quite stifling. It is not uncommon, moreover, for a person to feel that you are being violently attacked by this "entity." Being choked, being bitten, or having your limbs twisted are just a few of the sensations that people report.

The reader may be familiar with a famous painting by the British artist Henry Fuseli (1741-1825), called *The Nightmare* (1781), which shows a young woman lying on her bed, asleep, with a large hairy demon sitting on her chest. Floating above the foot of her bed is the ghostly head of a rather goofy-looking horse. The painting almost certainly depicts an SP attack. Was Fuseli an SP victim, I wonder? I wouldn't be surprised if he was, though I guess we'll never know.

As far as auditory hallucinations are concerned, the types of sounds and voices that SP sufferers hear vary widely. Buzzing, grinding, whirring, whistling, and ringing sounds are commonly reported. These are sometimes accompanied by strange bodily sensations, such as a tingling or numbness. Also reported are sounds of a "technological" nature. Siren noises and telephone noises are two typical examples.

Then there are the voices, some of them indistinct and unintelligible, others clear and comprehensible. For some strange reason, the latter are usually simple commands. Psychologist J. Allan Cheyne of the University of Waterloo (UW) in Canada, who, within the last decade or so, has collected in excess of 28,000 tales of SP, runs a popular SP webpage, from which I have obtained, for this book, numerous quotes by SP sufferers. On this webpage, one woman reported the following experience: "As I listened I could sense this 'thing' walk or hover over my head – very close directly over my ear. It said 'Freya!'...The voice continued: 'I've got work for you to do!' Then I listened as the presence hovered for a few seconds more and moved across the room to sit on my roommate's bed."

It's interesting to note that the sounds and voices people hear during

SP episodes are, for the most part, distinctly experienced as being external to the hearer, rather than thought-like and "in the head." Generally, they are not taken to be self-generated. In comparison to auditory hallucinations experienced during SP episodes, visual hallucinations are reported far less frequently and are often less vivid. The images people see are predominately indefinite and insubstantial. Often people see "shadowy" beings floating around the room or standing near the bed. Most of the entities I see are dark, shadowy serpentine creatures, with long, thrashing tails. I also see grey orbs of various sizes, which look like balls of liquid smoke. I will explain more about this later.

These days, SP is used to explain – and often unfairly dismiss – a significant number of nocturnal paranormal experiences, from alien abduction episodes to out-of-body experiences (OBEs). The phenomenon has had a profound impact on religion and mythology throughout the ages, not just in the West, but all over the world. Some have speculated that in medieval Europe, the belief in incubi and succubi, as well as other demons, and possibly even witchcraft, may have resulted from the SP phenomenon.

Although these days we refer to a nightmare as a fearful or disturbing dream, the meaning of the word has changed, and since around 1300 the word has been used in connection with the SP phenomenon. In England during the Middle Ages, to have a "nightmare" was to have an SP experience – an experience attributed to the influences of a "mare," a demonic being thought to attack people in the night, causing a sensation of pressure on the chest.

The mare – or mara – also exists in Scandinavian mythology and is described as a malignant female wraith. This immaterial being is believed to be capable of moving through a keyhole or the crack under a door. Once inside the victim's bedroom, she seats herself on their chest, then "rides" them. The sleeping victim is said to experience "nightmares" as a result.

Today, defined as having a worn or gaunt appearance through illness, lack of sleep, etc., the term "haggard" also relates to SP, for it was once believed that witches or hags attacked men in the night by riding on their chests as they slept. In Chinese folklore, SP is believed to be a form of minor body possession caused by forces of the dead, though it is said not to harm the victim in any real way. The Chinese name for SP translates as "ghost pressing on body," or "ghost pressing on bed."

References to SP-type phenomena can be found all over the world, in Japan, Thailand, Mexico, Greece, Indonesia, the Philippines, Hawaii, Russia, and Hungary. The list goes on. In most of these countries, spirits and other supernatural beings are thought to be behind SP episodes. Having had hundreds of SP experiences over the years, I can easily understand why this is the case. To become a victim of SP is to realize that invisible, non-physical beings do exist.

Apparently, it wasn't until the publication of David J. Hufford's groundbreaking 1982 book *The Terror That Comes in the Night* that researchers began to realize that SP affects the general population and is not exclusively a symptom of narcolepsy. Narcolepsy, as defined by *The American Heritage Dictionary*, "is a disorder characterized by sudden and uncontrollable, though often brief, attacks of deep sleep, sometimes accompanied by paralysis and hallucinations." It should be mentioned, too, that SP experiences differ from both night terrors and nocturnal panic attacks.

Some researchers make a distinction between the types of SP episodes experienced by the general population and those experienced by the narcoleptic population. In his book *Wrestling with Ghosts*, sleep researcher Jorge Conesa Sevilla sometimes uses the term Isolated Sleep Paralysis (ISP) to refer to the SP experiences of people "in otherwise normal populations without other symptoms, even when the SP experience is a once-in-a-life time event."

To say that SP is a subject about which there is much confusion would be putting it mildly. The fact that it was previously thought to be something that only narcoleptics suffered from is proof of this. And although it's beginning to gain acceptance as a fairly common condition, it remains little understood. So to help clarify matters, I need to stress the point that there are various forms of SP, such as SP accompanied by hypnagogic/hypnopompic hallucinations (sometimes called hypnagogic SP), and what one might term non-hypnagogic SP, or simply SP. If you were to undergo the latter type of episode, the only thing you would experience is bodily paralysis. There would be no hallucinations, and, most likely, the experience wouldn't leave much of an impression.

Some people, such as myself, experience episodes on a fairly regular basis and are sometimes referred to as chronic SP suffers. Others have episodes very infrequently – say every five years – and are therefore unlikely to think of themselves as having a disorder. The specific form of SP that I have – and which some alleged victims of alien abduction probably have also – is known as Recurrent Isolated Sleep Paralysis (RISP). RISP, as defined by Jean-Christophe Terrillon and Sirley Marques-Bonham in a paper published in the *Journal of Scientific Exploration*, "is a rarer variant of sleep paralysis characterized by frequent episodes or a complex of sequential episodes of generally longer duration, and in particular by the range and intensity of the perceptual phenomena occurring during episodes." Explained simply, RISP sufferers undergo, on a regular basis, generally long SP episodes, frequently accompanied by hypnagogic/hypnopompic hallucinations.

Although people are most likely to develop SP during their adolescent years – around the age of sixteen or seventeen – as happened to me, it is not uncommon to experience such episodes in childhood, nor is it impossible for a person to develop the condition at this age. I myself have vague memories of childhood SP episodes, some of them involving clear auditory hallucinations. I remember telling my brother when I was about six and he was about seven that "God" had spoken to me during the night. I was not asleep at the time, I insisted, but had just woken up. My brother said something to the effect of "Yeah, right!," and I quickly forgot the incident, only to remember it about ten years later, when I developed RISP in my teens. The incidence of SP tends to decline as people move into their twenties, becoming significantly lower after the age of around thirty.

The condition is thought to be hereditary because it's often shown to occur in families over many generations. This might explain why one of my uncles is, as far as I can determine, a chronic SP sufferer, as he claims to have had countless nocturnal visits from grey aliens and other entities. An artist of some note, my uncle is obsessed with fairly tale-type themes and frequently paints white rabbits dressed as people, gathered in the forest under the moonlight, surrounding nude, vulnerable girls. Some of these artworks remind one of *Alice in Wonderland*. Some of his other paintings feature fairies, cherubs, and other supernatural beings, many of them glowing.

Statistics for the prevalence of SP in the general population vary widely from study to study – depending, of course, in which country the study was conducted, how it was designed, what ages the participants were, and various other factors. Differing from the statistics mentioned earlier – that 25-to-40 percent of the population will undergo an SP episode at least once in the course of their life – are those provided by the 1990 *International Classification of Sleep Disorders* (*ICSD*), which states that the figure is 40-to-60 percent. On the University of Waterloo's SP webpage, the figure given is 25-to-30 percent. The *ICSD* further states that SP experiences are frequent in about 3-to-6 percent of the population. I ask, once again, that the reader bear in mind that not all SP experiences feature hallucinations, and that these statistics apply equally to those who see flying green goblins and have full-blown OBEs, as well as to those who experience nothing but short bouts of uncomfortable paralysis.

In a study carried out in 1999 by the American Academy of Neurology, which surveyed the sleeping habits of 8,100 German and Italian participants, nearly 30 percent of people with severe SP were found to experience hallucinations during their episodes. Taking these figures, as well as those provided by the *ICSD*, in concert, one can easily calculate the percentage of RISP sufferers (chronic SP sufferers who experience hallucinations) in the general population, which is 0.9-1.8 percent.

Not wanting to get bogged down in terminology, I will be using the term SP to refer to a whole range of such experiences, from those that involve hallucinations to some that don't. This seems to be the norm these days, anyway, with SP being used as a very broad term. Because, as explained in *The Abduction Enigma*, written by Kevin Randle, Russ Estes, and William Cone, "there is no single, simple definition of what sleep paralysis is," I feel it necessary to include a precise and comprehensive definition of the phenomenon, as given by R. J. Campbell in his dictionary of psychiatric terms:

"A benign neurological phenomenon, more probably due to some temporary dysfunction of the reticular activating system consisting of brief episodes of inability to move and/or speak when awakening or less commonly, when falling asleep. There is no accompanying disturbance of consciousness, and the subject has complete recall for the episode. The incidence of the phenomenon is highest in younger age groups (children and young adults) and much higher in males (80%) than females. It occurs in narcolepsy... The terms by which the phenomenon has been known are nocturnal hemiplegia, nocturnal paralysis, sleep numbness, delayed psychomotor awakening, cataplexy of awakening and post dormital chalastic fits."

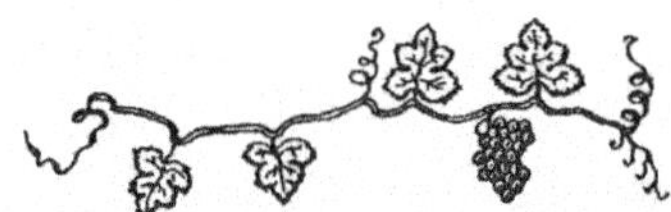

This book is an attempt to make sense of the SP phenomenon from an alternative, non-mechanistic perspective. Those of a skeptical disposition, who have little or no time for the occult or paranormal, will find nothing of value in this book. Only those who already have an interest in such subjects and are equipped with an open, but discerning, mind, are likely to enjoy this book and gain something from it. My hope is that SP sufferers like myself, who are fed up with the official explanation of SP, will find comfort within these pages and hopefully some answers, too.

Part one of *Dark Intrusions* deals primarily with the SP phenomenon and is rife with descriptions of my own SP episodes. Putting these experiences into words was by no means easy. When it comes to describing experiences of a paranormal nature – experiences that are of another realm and of another mode of consciousness – one is extremely limited by language. I ask that the reader bear this in mind. Please understand, moreover, that I am *not* recounting dreams, that what occurs during an SP episode goes far beyond anything that occurs during a dream and is a wholly different experience. If any of my SP experiences read like dreams, it's because I've failed to describe them adequately.

Part two of *Dark Intrusions* expands on what I deal with in part one, placing the subject of SP in a much broader context. Many of the topics explored in this section – among them, poltergeist disturbances, mediumship, channeling, alien abduction, Spiritism, OBEs, and shamanism – may strike the reader as largely unrelated, and one is likely to wonder what any of them have to do with SP. I can assure the reader, however, that there is a method in my madness. Had I not examined the SP phenomenon from as many different angles as possible, what I now know about the subject would be very limited indeed. Furthermore, it has long been my understanding that there is no subject in the paranormal/occult field that isn't related to another and which doesn't supplement another. Having a comprehensive knowledge of such matters allows one to recognize this truth.

I have to admit that much of what I've written herein has been colored – though not dogmatically so – by my interest in Spiritism, an offshoot of Spiritualism, which began in France in the mid-1800s. I make frequent references to two Spiritist texts – *The Spirits' Book* and *The Mediums' Book* – and quote extensively from them. Not until I'd finished writing *Dark Intrusions* did I realize that it had such a strong Spiritist flavor. I even felt compelled to include a chapter on Chico Xavier, Brazil's most famous Spiritist medium.

It would be accurate to say that this book, rather than being about SP, is essentially about the nature of incorporeal beings and the interactions that take place between them and us. I regard these matters as a kind of science – by no means a definite science, but a science nonetheless. It is my firm belief that we *can* bring the occult into the light, that what is classified as paranormal or supernatural need not remain elusive and incomprehensible.

One will notice, throughout the chapters of this book, a great many number of consistencies between the work of one paranormal researcher or shaman/occultist and that of another – consistencies that cannot be attributed to the sharing of information, or, for that matter, coincidence. These consistencies illuminate spiritual facts, and I think it is important that one takes notice of them. Only by piecing these facts together – rather than relying on purely subjective observations – can we begin to make any real progress with our understanding of the "spirit realm" and its inhabitants. It is my hope that this book is a step in the right direction.

PART 1

CHAPTER 1

"I Literally Fear For My Soul"

The year was 2001 and I was seventeen when my SP experiences began. I had previously been living with my father and brother in Tenterfield, New South Wales, in Australia, and had just moved down to Healesville, Victoria, to live with my mother. My new home was a Buddhist retreat center, where my mother worked as a caretaker. My room, no. 25, was located near the office and the main meditation hall. It was a reasonably small and humble room and, like most of those at the Buddhist center, would have suited a monk better than a teenager. Still, it was agreeable enough.

The year 2003, the year after I graduated from high school, was an idle period in my life. Events had taken a rather unfortunate turn, and my future did not look bright. I began to spend most of my days alone, reading in my bedroom with the curtains drawn, and occasionally writing in my journal. The activities I did to keep myself occupied were rarely ever constructive. I would start building something, a model plane, for example, suddenly become discouraged, and put the project aside, never to complete it. Whenever I felt nervous, stressed, or depressed, my SP experiences would become more frequent and more intense. Often, when life becomes unpleasant, one attempts to escape by finding comfort in sleep. But for me, that was becoming less possible.

It wasn't until mid-2007 that I fully recognized the fact that I suffered from SP. Ever since I first starting having episodes back in 2001, I had no idea what was happening to me. I had heard of the phenomenon before, but not enough to know anything substantial about it. At first, I worried obsessively about the state of my mental health. I even began to suspect that I might be developing schizophrenia, or some other serious and debilitating neurosis. When I did finally investigate the subject, I was both astonished and relieved to discover that other people had undergone, and were undergoing, the same bizarre experiences as me.

My SP experiences have changed over the years, gradually becoming more and more intense. They have now reached a kind of plateau, in that most of them are pretty much the same these days, and I know what to expect. Every now and then, however, I will have a particularly frightening or compelling episode, and I will not be able to forget it for a very long time – or at all. Instead of describing any single episode – of which there is only a handful that I remember with total clarity – I will attempt to shed light on what a typical episode involves. To do so, and in the most veracious way possible, it's necessary that I refer to a short story I wrote in 2005, during the first year of my diploma at RMIT University.

Written as an assignment for class, I gave it the rather sensational title "Beware of the Spirits who Feast on your Soul," and, although I didn't realize it then, the story relates directly to my SP experiences. Which is not to say, of course, that I had no idea what I was writing about at the time. I knew perfectly well what I was writing about – the bizarre and frightening experiences that were, and had been, happening to me at night; it's just that I did not have a label to assign to these experiences. Not wanting to have my mental health questioned, I gave no indication to either my classmates or my teacher that "Beware of the Spirits" was based on real experiences in my life.

What follows is an excerpt from "Beware of the Spirits." It's an accurate description of what I experience during a typical SP episode. The protagonist in the story, a teenage boy, is lying in bed, trying his hardest to get to sleep. He feels stressed and anxious. Frustrated that he cannot get to sleep or stop his mind from racing, he climbs out of bed and switches on the light. After listening to music for about half-an-hour, he attempts, once again, to go to sleep, and this time succeeds. It's then that things start to get interesting.

"After what seems like a short time later, I wake-up, but not completely. I can feel something touching my forehead; it is this that has drawn me kicking and screaming into a semi-conscious state. But in truth, I cannot kick or scream; in fact, I can't move a single muscle in my body, even though my mind is awake. For god's sake I can't even open my eyes. All I can do is lie there as this thing attends to my forehead with delicate, loving strokes. Whatever it is, I can smell the stench of its presence. I can taste its mind just as much as it can taste mine. But its love, its child-like affection, is sickening me, and all I want is for it to leave me in peace.

"I continue to lie there, engulfed by the darkness as the shadow strokes my forehead. It then moves over to the left side of my body and proceeds to lie down beside me. It writhes around annoyingly until it finds a comfortable position. Then, once it's finished messing around, it puts its arms around me. Its grip is so tight that my chest is aching. I want to scream out in fear and disgust, but there is nothing I can do.

"When it becomes too unbearable, I manage to find the strength inside myself to scream. It's only a faint scream, but it communicates the full extent of my rage. Right now, this is the only weapon I have. It's also a way of telling my assailant that I am not to be messed with. But in truth it's ridiculous, for the shadow is only encouraged by my raw expression of fear. Because fear is what it feeds on. And in response, as if in competition, the shadow screams as well. And its scream is far more powerful than mine; so powerful in fact, that it almost tears me apart.

"With greater strength than ever before, I force myself to wake-up by fighting the paralysis that grips my body. All the while, the shadow attempts to stop me by drawing me into the realm of sleep. But in the end I manage to break through. When I open my eyes and gaze around the pitch-black room, I see the shadow swirling above me, now in the form of a hideous, dark serpent. But I no longer fear it, for I am the victor in this battle. Now that I've woken up, it's powerless to hurt me.

"The shadow, I notice, looks vulnerable and weak. As it floats above me, it twists and flexes its body as if suffering from a fit. I repeatedly strike at its ghostly black form, but my hands pass straight through it. In defeat, the shadow floats up to the top of the ceiling and slithers across the underside of one of the rafters. Once it reaches the other side of the room, I lose sight of it amongst the shadows.

"I jump out of bed, switch on the light, and gaze around the room in an attempt to find the shadow. Just as I expected, it's nowhere to be found; it has returned to the ghostly realm from whence it emerged. I climb back in bed and try to collect my thoughts. I now know the shadow is well and truly gone, and this fills me with a sense of relief. I also know from experience that, even if it were to return, it would be incapable of reaching me while I'm awake. Which is why, for the time being, I decide not to drift back to sleep."

As the reader would have gathered from reading the above passage, SP experiences can be absolutely terrifying. Of all the episodes I've had over the years, about 90 percent of them were frightening to some degree. Fear plays a very significant role in the phenomenon, the main reason being that all SP attacks contain an element of helplessness. To quote again from "Beware of the Spirits": "I felt like a man who had been intentionally buried alive. I was trapped inside a dark, cramped coffin, thousands of meters underground, and my oxygen supply was running out quickly. And, to make matters worse, there was an evil, vicious thing outside, trying its hardest to penetrate the paper-thin walls surrounding me."

Apart from the fact that one is unable to move one's body and can sense a threatening presence nearby, there is another reason that these experiences generate so much fear, but it's difficult to put into words. One SP sufferer explained it best when they wrote, "I literally fear for my soul." The following comments, written by SP suffers, validate the blood curdling nature of the phenomenon:

- "The presence was of a demonic nature, purest evil, out to possess my soul . . . The presence was ALWAYS evil, and I could always feel it trying to enter my body . . . I find this utterly terrifying, beyond anything I can imagine experiencing in the real world because it is so contrary to 'reality', and yet feels entirely authentic . . . Not so much 'die,' more like losing possession of my soul."

- "The greatest primal terrors that I have ever witnessed: Character forming stuff – I can't imagine anything in reality that could cause greater fear than these episodes."

- "How about 'overwhelming terror?' These attacks leave me shuddering and crying. Sometimes I'm so scared I get sick to my stomach."

- "Fear is not a strong enough word! Terrified or panicked might be a better choice."

While in this aberrant state between wakefulness and sleep, there is usually nothing but total darkness inside one's mind. It's uncommon to see images in one's mind's eye. Sometimes, however, one is able to open one's eyes ever so slightly and may sense some movement. One might catch a glimpse of a translucent, ghostly form, leaning over one's body and moving so quickly that it's difficult to make out. Such has been the case in my experience – not just once, but on several occasions. Or, one may see a dark figure standing or floating in the bedroom, staring with piercing black eyes.

While struggling for freedom, trying hard to wake up and to fight the paralysis gripping one's body, one can not only sense the presence of the being that is trying to "possess" you, one can also "taste" its mind – just as I have described in the story. It feels as though the entity has managed to "lock onto" your very soul using a powerful suction cup. It's a very peculiar and highly unpleasant sensation. The word "rape" springs to mind. To be in total communion, in absolute mind-to-mind contact with another soul, is something that words fail to convey.

When I say that, during the SP state, one can "taste" the mind of the being that is attached to you, I mean exactly that. "Taste" is the best verb to use, though "smell" would also be suitable. Those of you who, like me, are highly intuitive and are sensitive to the vibes of people and places, would know exactly what I mean by this. The vibe of a person or place can sometimes be so powerful, I've noticed, that one can actually feel its radiation penetrate to the very core of one's being. In the SP state, one's soul is totally exposed, and no barrier exists to block your psychic impressions. In this peculiar state of consciousness, you are about a thousand times more sensitive to the psychic radiation emanating from people and places than when you are fully awake.

During the SP state, one is conscious of the fact that one possesses a "soul." One can sense, in other words, that your mind exists independently of your physical body, and that the former is secondary in importance to the latter. One can also sense that your being has an energy body of its own. This non-physical body is commonly known as the astral body. My research seems to indicate that the majority of SP attacks occur on an astral level, and that the SP state involves a partial dislocation of the astral body from the physical body. According to many occultists, the astral body leaves the physical body regularly during the sleep state, while dreams are often memories of the astral journeys we take. We will explore this theory in far greater depth, once we come to the work of the late Robert Monroe, an expert on OBEs.

In my experience, the sensations of the astral body are very different from those experienced by the physical body. For instance, the "hand" of a spirit feels slightly synthetic, almost rubbery, but in no way lifeless. "Spirit skin" feels nothing like human skin. In "Beware of the Spirits," I described what it's like to feel the touch of spirits. One time I felt a pair of hands around my neck, as a rather vicious being tried to choke me to death. I honestly thought I was going to die. During less sinister, even pleasant, encounters, I have felt the tiny playful hands of spirits touch me on the chest, side, and shoulders. I could sense they meant me no harm.

In "Beware of the Spirits," the protagonist is attacked twice by a powerful, invisible entity. I have already mentioned the first attack. The following is a description of the second attack, which, it should be remembered, was written at a time when I was almost completely ignorant of the SP phenomenon.

"Once again, I half wake-up and my body is entirely paralyzed. As usual, I can feel and sense a presence nearby. This time the shadow is sitting at the end of my bed, and the weight of its body is crushing my legs. Unlike the previous night, I decide not to wake myself up, as I'm curious to know what the shadow will do next. As if in response to my thoughts, the shadow slithers closer. Now I can hear and feel its warm breath on my face. This sensation, both irritating and sickening, reminds me that the shadow is a living, breathing creature, and not at all a figment of my imagination.

"The shadow crawls across my stomach, closer to my face. I feel a curious sensation as it attaches something to my mind. To have my mind touched, prodded, almost tickled, is a feeling that words fail to describe. All I know is that my mind is being violated, as nothing has ever gotten so close to my soul. But still, out of burning curiosity, I let the shadow continue. Now I can hear the shadow's voice in my head: 'For a long time I've waited for this moment.' I let these words echo in my head, so that I have a chance to taste the shadow's essence. Surprisingly, its voice is nothing like what I expected; it's clear, polite, almost robotic, and not at all sinister."

In my story, I describe sensing an evil presence nearby. This experience, called the "sensed presence," is a common aspect of the SP phenomenon. Sometimes one feels that the presence is trying to take over or invade one's mind, or is attempting to steal one's very soul. According to one SP sufferer, "There is usually always an intense feeling of extreme evil surrounding me. I also feel a presence in my mind (like something sinister or evil) that is trying to draw me into an extremely deep, permanent sleep. I feel that if I succumb, I will never wake up."

Sometimes, during the SP state, I also feel that my attacker "is trying to draw me into an extremely deep, permanent sleep," and that, if I let myself succumb, I will not be able to wake up, perhaps even die. I have described this feeling in "Beware of the Spirits." Here are those words again: "With greater strength than ever before, I force myself to wake-up by fighting the paralysis that grips my body. All the while, the shadow attempts to stop me by drawing me into the realm of sleep. But I manage to break through."

"I manage to break through," means I manage to wake up, which, by the way, can be one hell of a struggle. Imagine you're underwater, with lead weights attached to your feet, and you're trying to swim to the surface, but the weight keeps dragging you down. That's what it feels like. The reason I manage to "break through to the surface," so to speak, and have on every occasion, is because of my powerful will to survive – which is something we all possess.

When confronted by a dangerous, life-threatening situation, one is often able to draw on enormous reserves of energy. We've all heard those remarkable tales of survival, whereby, following an accident, people have managed to lift cars off the bodies of their loved ones. The same rule applies to the SP phenomenon. Believe me, when you feel that your soul is being stolen by the devil himself, you will not take a passive approach. On the contrary, you will fight as hard as you can to resist, and you will not give up.

Featured in the second half of "Beware of the Spirits" is a good description of this feeling. The protagonist has just emerged from a nightmare, in which the "shadow" made an appearance, and has now entered the SP state. The entities responsible for SP episodes are, by the way, able to invade one's dreams, turning them into nightmares. I will explain this aspect of the phenomenon later on.

"Suddenly, something flashed inside my mind, and I realized I was dreaming, that none of this was entirely real. Right then, I desired nothing more than to wake up. I had to get out of this evil place. I had to evade the demon who was trying to capture my soul. For some reason I felt that he was the only real part – the only real danger – of the nightmare I was struggling to escape from. And so, I kept trying to wake myself up. I pushed hard against the invisible barrier that separates the world of dreams from the world of physical reality. I used every ounce of strength that I possessed. After making a small amount of progress, I could tell that my physical senses were starting to come back. My body, in other words, was gradually returning to a state of sensation and control.

"Although the world inside my head was dark, and I couldn't see, I could sense that the shadow was close by. It was trying to draw me back into the world of sleep – where it normally dwelt – so that it could consume me. With ever increasing force, it was attempting to take possession of my mind and body. Determined not to give in – although it was tempting – I kept up the struggle. As I fought harder, I gained more awareness – both physically and mentally. And, after a short while, I was conscious of the fact that I was lying in bed. However, I was still unable to move my body, or, for that matter, see; all around me there was only darkness – a darkness that stretched on for eternity. But this darkness was not without life..."

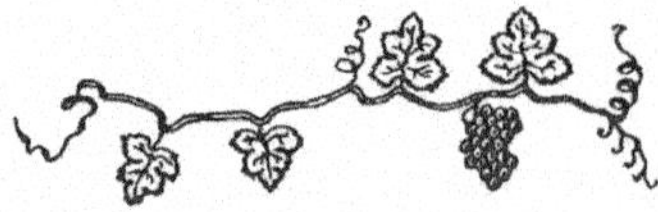

During the year 2003, the SP experiences I was having were rather unique. Some of them, I'm almost embarrassed to admit, were of a highly sexual nature. Unbelievable though it sounds, I had sexual intercourse with female spirits who visited me in the middle of the night. This happened on several occasions. These sexual encounters were generally very intense; in many ways, more so than the real thing. What I experienced was similar to, but not quite the same as, "real" sex. These encounters would always take place in a quasi-SP state, slightly different from the normal SP state.

I now know there is a great deal of truth to the medieval stories of succubi and incubi attacks. The incubus and its female counterpart, the succubus, are demonic beings that, during medieval times, were believed to be responsible for attacking people who slept. The male incubus, which mainly preyed on women, was said to lie on top of its victims in order to have sexual intercourse with them.

According to folklore, when a succubus or incubus wishes to seduce someone, they alter their appearance in such a way as to appear more sexually appealing and more humanoid. Their true form is that of a typical-looking demon, with horns, bat-like wings and a pointy tail. They are vampires who feed off the energy of their victims in order to sustain themselves. Following an attack, the victim can be so exhausted, so drained of vital energy, that death may result. Legend has it that succubi would collect semen from the men they slept with, which incubi would then use to impregnate women.

One cannot help but be reminded of modern day alien abduction stories, involving the collection of sperm from men and the artificial impregnation of women. Fairies, elves, and other mythological beings, not unlike today's greys, also took an active interest in such matters. How does one explain this preoccupation with human reproduction by beings not of this world?

Sex with spirits and demons is not an uncommon phenomenon. Encounters of the sort have been recorded since at least the Middle Ages and have probably been going since time immemorial. While it would be easy to dismiss such stories as nothing more than the fantasies of the sexually starved and the sexually repressed, it would seem that the truth is far stranger.

Of all the succubi encounters I've had over the years, there is one in particular that I remember as clear as day. Interestingly, the being who straddled me didn't seem to know what she was doing. Instead of it being a smooth, rhythmic process, as is normally the case, the experience was particularly awkward. As I was lying on my back comfortably and, I admit, quite happily, she was having a very challenging time on top.

In comparison to ordinary sex, "spirit sex" is certainly far more intense, being more of an internal process than an external one. One's entire being is permeated by a feeling of total and absolute pleasure. One might describe it as a merging of two souls, of two energies with opposite polarities, which, when combined, complement and galvanize each other. I have described the beings I encountered as "female spirits," not succubi, because they did not appear to be vampiric and/or demonic in any way. Not once have I felt drained of energy following an encounter of this sort. Most of them were quite pleasant, even if a little strange.

During one encounter, I managed to open my eyes ever so slightly while the experience was taking place. I was rather taken aback to discover that the female being on top of me had the appearance of a half-human, half-alien grey. She was tall and skinny, with legs like long stilts. Her body was slightly translucent, as though she were a ghost. Putting it the politest way possible, I would have to say she was not my type. I've never fancied women with grey skin and bug-like eyes!

CHAPTER 2

Strange Hallucinations

At the start of 2004, I relocated from the peaceful town of Healesville to the noisy inner-city suburb of Carlton North. Much in my life had changed by then, though my SP experiences continued. I had always thought that the Buddhist center was in some way haunted, that the supposed ghosts inhabiting the place were the ones responsible for attacking me in the night, and that, if I moved away, my experiences would become less severe, or would cease altogether. How wrong I was.

The place I moved into was another Buddhist center. (The centre in Healesville and the one in Carlton were owned by the same group of Buddhists.) My new bedroom was dusty, dark, and had once been used as a laundry. It had a very unpleasant atmosphere. Sticking out of the walls were numerous metal pipes, the taps removed from the ends. In one corner of the room was a large concrete slab about a foot high, which, as far as I could determine, had once served as a platform for washing machines and basins. Although the room was by no means perfect, it was in a convenient location, and the rent was cheap. I was reasonably happy with it.

It was around this time that I began to experience auditory hallucinations, not while awake, thank god, but during the SP state. This would have to be one of the most frightening aspects of the phenomenon that I've had to deal with. There is something deeply unsettling about hearing a foreign voice outside (or inside) your head. It's a horrible intrusion into the private territory of one's soul. I have already explained that the auditory hallucinations of SP sufferers, rather than being internal, are generally experienced in such a fashion as to give one the impression that the sound is coming from outside oneself.

On one occasion, while sleeping peacefully and having a pleasant dream, I felt something "lock onto" my mind. I identified the sensation immediately, realizing that it was the beginning of an SP attack. A split second later, I heard a thundering voice shout directly in my ear, "Why do you want to leave this place?" The voice was that of an American hillbilly. It was strange and very foreign and did not sound like anyone I knew, or had ever heard before, either in a film or TV show. I cannot overemphasize the overwhelmingly real and convincing nature of the voice, as being not a creation of my own mind, but as something produced by an intelligence from "out there," in no way connected to myself.

To say the voice startled me would be an understatement; it scared the absolute hell out of me, waking me up instantly. I jumped out of bed and switched on the light, my body trembling in shock. I was angry at the damn hillbilly who had rudely woken me up. I wanted to throttle the scoundrel – I was that mad. Walking back to bed, I could sense a distinct presence, watching me with interest, in the corner of the room.

In fact, before I'd turned on the light, I thought I saw a luminous, smoky substance hovering in the very same area, just above my bed, though I'm willing to admit that it may have been a product of my imagination. After all, not everything one sees, hears, etc, during the SP state, or the hypnagogic/hypnopompic state, can be attributed to spirits and the like. Sometimes it's simply nonsense, nothing more nothing less, and should be identified as such. Those who have frequent SP episodes learn to distinguish the real from the imaginary.

Was the voice a product of my unconscious mind? A question worth considering, but I highly doubt it. I do not see why my unconscious mind (however one might define it), would want to wake me (my conscious mind) up by asking a cryptic question at two in the morning. What would be the point of it?

The reader is probably wondering what the aforementioned question related to, if anything at all. Fortunately, I'm able to shed some light on the matter. At that time in my life, I had just been given notice to vacate the room in which I was lodging. The matter was resting heavily on my mind, for I had been staying in the room for more than three years, had become attached to it, and was feeling anxious about having to search for a new place to stay. I was in two minds about the idea, my thoughts shifting often from the positive to the negative. At the time I was asked this question, my opinion on the matter was a positive one. I was feeling sick of my current home, due to its overwhelming familiarity, and was looking forward to a change. I have a strong feeling that the question, "Why do you want to leave this place?" related to this event in my life.

It's interesting to note that the question sounded so casual, as though the being who asked it was a friend of mine, and we were having a relaxed conversation. It reminded me of an incident that occurred many years ago, when I was fifteen years old and travelling on a bus from Melbourne to Tenterfield, a journey of about 24 hours. It was early in the morning and I was sleeping lightly, when suddenly I was awoken by a man seated behind me with a loud, obnoxious voice, who thought I should know that we were stopping for breakfast in twenty minutes. He shouted the words in my ear and obviously had little regard for common manners. The "spirit voice" that woke me up was much the same. Whoever or whatever was behind it didn't seem to be conscious of the fact that it's impolite to rouse someone, unless, of course, there's a good reason for doing so.

In my case – and I suspect this is true of most SP sufferers – I will usually hear voices and sounds during the final moments of an SP episode, never at the beginning, and rarely during the middle. Why this is, I do not know for sure, although I suspect it has something to do with being in the exact right state of consciousness for the phenomenon to be possible.

It's common for SP sufferers to forget the voices they've heard shortly after waking up. Such has been the case in my experience, though I have managed to remember a few statements, one of them being the question just mentioned. Why it is that most of the things I've been told, or asked, were cryptic in nature is anybody's guess. This seems to be the case with many of the voices SP sufferers hear. Are the beings behind the voices deliberately trying to confuse us? On the University of Waterloo's SP webpage, one individual wrote: "I heard a voice telling me I was playing the game wrong and I had to play it right or quit. It was a woman's voice and she sounded as though she were in a lot of pain and very far away, then she said, he's coming and left."

The following experience, from Sevilla's *Wrestling with Ghosts*, was reported by a twenty-four-year-old male known as JB: "I heard a male voice and it was coming from the ceiling and it said, 'It's time to play games now.'...The other voice during another episode was a female voice and it said, 'What are you going to do (JB)." When I first read these words, it sent a shiver down my spine, because it reminded me of some of the SP voices I've heard. Believe me when I say that the spirits responsible for SP attacks are dirty, rotten scoundrels, the absolute lowest of the low. They will do anything they can to induce fear in their victims and will say the creepiest things imaginable.

More often than not, the voice will be unintelligible or indistinct. Sometimes it seems that whoever is behind the voice is situated on the other side of the room, or is whispering, or is not "tuned in" properly. I have used the words "tuned in" for a very important reason, because it seems to me that when a spirit wishes to communicate with a person telepathically, the process is similar to that of finding the right station, the right frequency, on a radio dial.

When the being behind the attack is firmly "locked on" to one's mind, which, as I've explained, is something that can be felt, then the voice one hears will be clear and loud. In this instance, "reception" is good, the station being "tuned in" just right. On the other hand, when the voice one hears is faint and indistinct, and appears to come from far away, it means the "station" has not been tuned in correctly. This is a minor SP attack – the kind of attack that can be easily "shaken off." *When an incorporeal being wishes to establish communication with a person, the process is one of correct tuning.*

According to one SP sufferer, "I sometimes hear people (who I think are in the room talking), or music that I think my family or friends are playing." Another individual reported the following: "Usually the sounds are that of people talking or yelling outside. Sometimes it will be a familiar voice like that of my mother. Usually unfamiliar. Many times I will hear high pitched noises, very loud, usually increasing if I don't wake up."

That this individual said the voices get louder the longer they remain in the SP state strikes me as very interesting because it's something I've experienced a number of times. It's interesting, too, because it brings us back to the radio analogy. Let me explain. While one is in the SP state, there is a very definite feeling of being "dragged under," of being possessed to a more and more extreme degree. On one occasion, as an experiment, I decided not to resist the experience. When I did this, when I let my mind drift for a second or two, my attacker was able to place an even firmer grip on my mind. Consequently, the voice I heard became even louder. During the brief moment that I yielded to the attack, my attacker was able to "tune in" easily – hence the clearer "reception," or louder voice.

Sounds of people moaning, screaming, and laughing are also reported by SP sufferers. During a typical SP episode – these days, anyway – I will almost always hear a clear and comprehensible voice address me directly. One time, as related in "Beware of the Spirits," I heard a male robotic voice; it was robotic in the sense that it sounded as though a machine produced it. It was unlike any electronically generated voice I have ever heard before. I've heard the voices of old men, old women, teenagers, middle-aged people, and, as I've already mentioned, hillbillies and "robots" as well. Each one is very distinctive. Some of them – at least two – are recurring. Why it is that some of the voices are recurring, while the rest of them I hear but once, is something I've often puzzled over.

Of the majority of the voices I've heard so far, their tone could best be described as intelligent, sophisticated, smug, and a little smart-alecky. Perhaps somewhat regrettably, I hardly ever get the chance to hear what they're trying to tell me. Out of fear of being totally possessed, and probably rightly so, I always wake myself up before they get the opportunity to make themselves heard, and will usually only catch the first three words of whatever it is I'm being told. Most of the voices speak in such a way that it seems they're trying to tell me something of great importance, something that requires my full attention. But, once again, the fear of being possessed overrides my curiosity every single time. Some of the voices come across as very annoying, and I can tell they have nothing of value to say, but are simply babbling on, talking for the sake of talking, like drunken idiots at a bar.

When an abject spirit realizes it's able to make contact with a human being, or is able communicate through a human being, it jumps at the opportunity with the enthusiasm of a ravenous dog. It desperately wants to be heard. And if its human victim happens to be in the SP state – which is a fairly vulnerable and delicate state of consciousness – then so be it; they're just as good as a medium, if not better, because an experienced medium has a reasonable amount of control over that which is temporarily "possessing" their body, whereas an SP sufferer has very little. The latter is defenseless and exploitable. The relationship between the SP phenomenon and mediumship is something I will elucidate at the appropriate time. Suffice it to say that the state of consciousness of a medium in trance, and that of someone in the SP state, is very similar in frequency.

SP suffers not only hear voices but strange sounds as well. SP sufferers report all types of mysterious sounds, but they tend to fall into several broad categories, of which, according to the University of Waterloos's SP webpage, there are three – elementary, technological, and natural. Belonging in the first category are the following types of sounds: buzzing, grinding humming, ringing, roaring, rushing, screeching, squeaking, vibrating, whirring, and whistling. According to psychologist Allan Cheyne, these elementary sounds "are often described as being very loud and 'mechanical,'" and "are sometimes accompanied by bodily sensations described as 'tingling,' 'numbness,' or 'vibration.'" One SP sufferer reported hearing "a high, humming sound that gets louder and louder the further I fall into the 'trance.'"

"On one occasion," wrote another SP sufferer, "I heard pure tones of sound, but it wasn't music. It was very erratic and unorganized." Interestingly, many people describe the sounds they hear as more of a vibration than anything else. "It's not exactly a sound," wrote one individual. "I felt a vibration inside my head that produced a noise." Another person described what they experienced as being "more of a bodily buzzing and swirling."

I should mention, at this point, that elementary sounds, and sensations of vibration and the like, do not feature strongly in my SP episodes. Only once or twice have I experienced a feeling of vibration; the last time, as of writing this, was in mid-2007. The sensation was most unusual and a little uncomfortable, almost unpleasant. As I lay there, totally paralyzed, I felt the vibrations throb throughout my body, from my head to my feet, permeating every fiber of my being. The energy seemed to pulse back and forth at a specific frequency. And, I discovered to my amazement, I was able to alter the frequency of the pulsations simply by willing them to change. Robert Monroe describes a similar phenomenon in *Journeys Out of the Body*.

SP sufferers report a range of strange bodily sensations. One said, "Right as it starts, I feel like I am being electrocuted slowly." And another wrote: "My whole body felt like it was vibrating inside at some incredible rate. I was afraid that my body and my brain would not physically be able to stand it. I also felt a numbness and electrical vibration, and would feel stuck to my bed."

What of technological sounds? "There is always a siren-like screeching that gets louder and louder, and some nights it's almost unbearable," wrote one SP sufferer. Another SP sufferer reported two main recurrent sounds. "One is like air entering a vacuum; it happens sometimes when entering or leaving the [SP] state as the ears become functional again. *The other sound is like a radio being heard from another room in the house. Many stations at the same time; barely intelligible*" (my emphasis). Another individual described the sound they heard as "like high pitched power tools...drills or band-saws that were close to my ears and gained in volume and intensity until I felt like my head was going to explode."

As for "natural" sounds, one of the most common is that of rushing air or wind. One SP sufferer described it as "a shrill, whistling sound – sound of 'wind.'" Another person wrote: "I felt I was in a sandstorm. I could hear the wind and sand rushing past my ears with a loud (sound) gust of wind." Other natural sounds include "a rushing/roaring sound like waves in a sea shell, almost or maybe similar to white noise." Could some of these sounds, I wonder, be attributed to perfectly natural causes? The answer is yes. Some of them could easily be real sounds that the mind has distorted in some way. The wind-like sounds, for instance, were possibly caused by exactly that – the wind.

Belonging in the natural sounds category are sounds of movement and animal sounds. "A commonly reported sound is that of footsteps," explains

Cheyne. On the University of Waterloo's SP webpage, one individual wrote that they often hear someone walking around their apartment, yet they live alone. The sound of footsteps – which is something I've heard during many an SP episode – pops up again and again. "There was a sound rather like a cardboard box or some weight being dragged across a dusty, wooden floor," wrote another SP sufferer.

Let us now move on to animal sounds, which I've heard on several occasions. These, mind you, were not your usual animal sounds. Whatever "creatures" were responsible for the noises I heard were certainly not of this world. To put it mildly, they sounded like beings from hell. In "Beware of the Spirits" I described an incident that occurred some years ago, in which I screamed in fear, and my attacker screamed as well, "…as if in competition…And its scream is far more powerful than mine; so powerful in fact, that it almost tears me apart."

On the University of Waterloo's SP webpage, one individual wrote, "I have heard 'growls' like a dog from hell or some other monster." When I first read these words, I was astonished because they describe, perfectly, the exact quality of the growls I heard. There must be more than a few "dogs from hell" roaming the realm of the astral. Or maybe we encountered the same one! Whatever the case may be, it was a very aggressive beast, I can tell you that. Although I joke about the experience now, it was no laughing matter when it occurred. To describe that demonic growl as the epitome of evil would be an understatement. It was pure, unadulterated malevolence. It struck fear into the very core of my being, almost shattering my soul. I hope to god that I never hear it, or anything like it, ever again.

Let us now address the topic of visual hallucinations. There are two main hallucinatory states associated with sleep – hypnagogic and hypnopompic. Hypnagogic hallucinations precede sleep, occurring while one is in a drowsy state of mind. They are more likely to occur than hypnopompic hallucinations, and, as a result, have been more extensively studied. Hypnopompic hallucinations, on the other hand, precede waking. Because the majority of SP attacks occur shortly after waking up, SP sufferers are more likely to experience the latter than the former. There appears to be little variance, if any at all, between the hallucinations one experiences in the hypnagogic state and those one experiences in the hypnopompic state.

I know several people who have had hypnagogic hallucinations, and who, to my astonishment, were rather reluctant to talk about their experiences for fear of being seen as crazy. If only they realized that these experiences are common to a significant portion of the population and are actually quite "normal." It's possible, in fact, for one to induce hypnopompic hallucinations at will, though it does take a certain amount of practice.

Some time ago, while hanging out a pub with a group of friends, I ended up having a fascinating conversation with a man, who, like me, had an interest in "altered states of consciousness." I will call him Frank. During the course of our conversation, I broached the subject of my SP experiences. I told Frank about the frightening voices, the strange serpentine creatures I had seen floating around my bedroom, and so on. Not wanting to appear totally insane, however, I omitted certain details of my experiences.

About halfway through the conversation, Frank began to open up about his own hallucinatory experiences. He told me he had hypnagogic hallucinations on a regular basis and had, over the years, seen some very peculiar things – spiders in particular, for some reason. I asked him why this was so, and he told me he had no idea. He certainly did not suffer from arachnophobia – of that he was quite adamant. He was neither scared of spiders, nor was he especially comfortable around them. For him, spiders held no special significance, yet they kept reappearing in his hallucinations. He saw other things too. One evening, he said, while lying in bed, relaxing, he saw "a woman's head float into the room and drift out again." She appeared to be laughing.

For some strange reason, spiders feature heavily in accounts of hypnopompic/hypnagogic hallucinations. One time, after I had just woken up, I saw a spider dangling from a silver cord just above my head. It was shiny, black and metallic, and looked entirely real and solid. I even saw it move; it did so in a very mechanical fashion, extending and contracting its metallic legs. Thinking it was real, I crawled out of bed, keeping my head low so as to avoid making contact with it. Once out of bed, I turned around and noticed the spider had vanished into thin air – all in the period of a split second. It was then that I realized it was only a hallucination.

What's particularly interesting about my spider hallucination was the very convincing nature of it. For the most part, hypnopompic/hypnagogic hallucinations of the visual kind have an indefinite, insubstantial quality. Very rarely does one see clear, well-defined images and is taken in by them.

One can usually tell that the images are not entirely real. "The visual imagery of SP often appear to be less substantial than normal perception," explains Cheyne, "but are clearly taken to be perceived in external space," and lie "somewhere between full hallucinations and pseudo-hallucinations."

On one occasion, wrote one SP sufferer, "I felt...a presence, and saw a kind of specter. It was a misty form floating above my feet, and I felt that it was the cause of my discomfort." Another SP sufferer woke up to find "what I thought was a man leaning over me in bed, who had my right arm in a tight grip, holding me down on the bed...I was frozen for what seemed like forever, staring up into his face. The room was dark and the face was in shadows, so I mostly saw an outline of the face. When at last I could move, I whispered 'What do you want?' and the face seemed to just disappear into the flowered pattern of my bedroom drapes."

One of the most recent visual hallucinations I've had was of an alien grey standing right beside my bed, its entire body heavily obscured by shadow. I was lying down at the time, and had just woken up. The being's head, I recall, was at the same level as mine, so I was able to stare right into his face. Its dark eyes were moist and slightly reflective. Before I opened my eyes and saw the "alien," I was in a light SP state, and I felt it grab me by the hand, ever so lightly. The being's hand was tiny and soft, like that of a child's. It lingered in the room for several seconds before vanishing into thin air.

Although I refer to the "alien" as a hallucination, I'm quite sure it was in some sense real, but obviously not in a physical way. Being in an altered state of consciousness, my perception was able to reach into that mysterious other realm I have already mentioned – the astral realm. That the "alien" touched me before I woke up and saw it, seems to add credibility to the experience – credibility in the sense that what I saw is less likely to have been a product of my imagination.

My most impressive visual hallucination to date took place on May 15, 2008, in the early hours of the morning. Prior to emerging in the SP state, I had been having some very odd dreams – not especially frightening, just strange and out of place. Having drifted into a deep SP state – a state, that is, in which I felt barely conscious – I became aware of a presence near the end of the bed. From what I could gather by "reading its mind," the presence was neither human nor elemental, but something entirely different. It appeared to be part-human, part-elemental.

I use the term "elemental" to refer to a particular type of incorporeal entity, a kind of territorial animal whose actions are largely instinctive. The complexity and intelligence of these entities varies. Most elementals are really quite harmless. They're like dogs, but, thank god, without sharp teeth. Over the years, I've had numerous encounters with these beings and will explain more about them shortly.

As I tried to determine what the entity was, and what it wanted from me, the SP state in which I was in became much lighter. I was now able to think clearly and felt entirely awake, though of course my body remained paralyzed. I could sense that the entity was harmless enough, and that it regarded me with intense curiosity, as though it were meeting a human for the very first time. A moment later, I could feel the entity sitting on my solar plexus; its weight was equivalent to that of a small cat. It began moving around a great deal, occasionally kicking its long legs into the air.

I tried ignoring the entity, but it wouldn't leave me alone. It shifted closer, sitting down at a spot on my left side, not that far from my head. I decided to remain calm and in control, and not give in to my fear. I found I could open my eyes and even turn my neck ever so slightly. My bedroom was very dark, although there was a small amount of moonlight shining through a crack in the curtain, some of which was striking the entity, illuminating its hideous face, which I was able to see out of the corner of my eye.

With its large, wrinkled head and glassy, black eyes, the entity resembled some sort of troll. Its facial expression was one of self-satisfaction. Still paralyzed, I lay there studying it for a moment, until suddenly it noticed that I was staring at it and turned its head towards me. The entity looked startled, embarrassed even, for it must have assumed I was sound asleep. What happened next is difficult to put into words. The entity rose into the air, began shrinking, then vanished as if it were being sucked down a tube. The entire process happened in a couple of seconds, probably less.

What impressed me most about the encounter was the overwhelming realness of the entity. It looked like a part of objective reality and in no way hallucinatory. I'll never forget the look it gave me. I received the distinct impression that the entity was surprised that I noticed it. That it "fled" when it did seems to indicate that it did not want to be seen. Did I really hallucinate this creature, this ugly troll, into existence? Was it solely a product of my mind? My feeling is that it wasn't, and that it existed independently of my own mind.

Fortunately, not all the visual hallucinations I've had could be classified as frightening. Some of them, in fact, have been quite fun and humorous. There is one in particular that springs to mind. On the night it happened,

I found myself in a very light SP state, a warm, delicate trance. I soon became aware of a presence nearby, hovering around my body. Because I was tired and wanted to be left in peace, I tried telling it, using my mind, to annoy someone else. I could tell it meant me no harm and was only "goofing around." It was simple, unintelligent, though very mischievous, and must have belonged to the elemental category.

Throughout the night, it kept tapping me on the upper-half of my body, particularly on my shoulders. It began to get quite irritating. I tried ignoring the damn thing, but it was no use. Using what felt like a giant hand, it gave me one final tap on the shoulder. Actually, it was more of a slap. It used more force this time, and I woke up instantly.

What I saw next was very interesting. Floating in the air, a couple of feet from my face, was a large, translucent hand – a sort of ghostly hand but with well-defined edges and three-dimensions. It had a beautiful blue luminosity about it. I couldn't take my eyes off it. Instantly, the hand began to move. It extended and retracted its fingers in a smooth, graceful motion. Rather than looking like a separate part of the human body, however, it looked like a living thing in itself. As though filled with helium, the hand began to rise into the air. Before finally disappearing, it waved at me, as if to say goodbye, in the most kind and charming way.

For about a year, while I was still living at the Buddhist centre in the city, there was one particular type of entity that I kept seeing again and again, and which, fortunately, I haven't seen since. I would classify it as a type of energy parasite. Of all the different types of entities I've encountered over the years, it would have to be among the most dangerous. I use the word "dangerous" for a very good reason because I'm sure this creature is capable of causing serious harm to its victims, particularly if they're already in a low energy state and suffering from an illness, for example. The creature I speak of is dark in color and shaped like a large leech. It looks and behaves like an animal.

I've been attacked by this, or these, ghastly creatures several times, and I hope to god that it never happens again. My story "Beware of the Spirits" describes an encounter with one of these beings, "a hideous, dark serpent." To say that the creature looked like a "serpent" is not entirely accurate, however, as it more accurately resembled a "leech." The creature moved in a serpentine fashion, twisting and flexing its body a great deal, but it did not look like a serpent. Please excuse the inaccuracy in my story. On those few occasions when I saw these beings, I had just woken up, following an SP attack, and was in the hypnopompic state. My eyes were wide open.

The type of SP attack caused by these energy parasites is particularly frightening and overwhelming. They are, after all, very powerful beings, capable of depleting your vital energy to a life-threatening degree. You are placed under a spell so powerful that you fear that you will never wake up. Also, you are likely to feel a strong sensation of something latching onto your head. It's a kind of sucking sensation, such as that caused by a vacuum cleaner nozzle attached to the skin. In addition to this, you will sometimes feel what seems like cold air blowing against your face. You will notice that the "air" appears to be issuing from the mass attached to your head, as it presumably expands and contracts, like an octopus. While this is taking place, you can taste the cold animal mind of your attacker, in all its metallic bitterness.

Following the attack, you will see, usually right above your head, one of the leach-type creatures just described – sometimes several of them, often of various sizes. Their bodies have a shadowy, insubstantial appearance. While the hypnopompic state lasts, and perception is possible, you are able to interact with these creatures. On several occasions, I've tried to scare them off, and keep them at bay, by thrashing my arms around wildly – and it's actually worked; they've responded as threatened animals would. They are, I've discovered, quite cowardly and will often flee to the other side of the room or become extremely agitated.

As soon as I leave the hypnopompic state, the creatures vanish. But the fear they've inflicted can remain for quite some time – so much so, that I'll be too scared to go back to sleep straight away and will stay up for several hours, trying to calm myself. When I wake up the following morning – usually much later than intended – I will feel totally lethargic, like a zombie. It's a horrible sensation, of not just feeling drained of energy but of feeling defiled and unclean, too, almost like a rape victim.

It usually takes me a whole day to get my energy back and to center my mind again. In "Beware of the Spirits," I described what this highly unpleasant condition is like: "I feel physically and mentally drained from the night before, and it shows when I examine my face in bathroom mirror. I notice that my eyes are unusually red, while my hair is messier than ever – this proves that I've been tossing and turning in bed all night, due to the shadow's assault on my mind."

The reason I've spent so much time describing the characteristics of these entities, and not other types of entities, is because I'm so well acquainted with them. There are somewhere around 18,000 different species of fish living in the sea, and I'm sure there must be as many different species of entities inhabiting the astral realm. On several occasions, I've spotted strange jellyfish-like creatures floating leisurely around my bedroom, their bodies expanding and contracting in a hypnotic rhythm. They seemed entirely harmless.

I've seen other types of creatures, too. I mentioned having seen mysterious orbs of dark, smoky energy hovering in the air near my bed. These entities are fascinating to look at, especially at close range. Covering their "bodies" is a kind of watery skin, giving them the appearance of soap bubbles filled with smoke. If one were to look closely at the skin of a soap bubble one would notice how it moves ever so slowly, as though rotating. The orbs I've seen had this exact same quality – their skins were able to move. Interesting, too, is that there appears to be a field of subtle radiation surrounding these entities, a kind of aura.

Those of you familiar with the spirit orb phenomenon that's been sweeping the internet of late would probably suspect that I've been looking at alleged photographs of orbs, and that these images have colored my hypnopompic experiences. I can assure you that this is not the case. I have been seeing these entities for a long time now, well before the orb phenomenon hit the internet. Of course, many photographs of alleged spirit orbs can be explained by the presence of ambient light, or the light emitted by a flash, reflecting off dust particles or water droplets in the air in front of the camera, the image distorted by the camera's unfocused CCD lens. Some images, however, cannot be so easily dismissed. There have been orb photographs taken, for instance, where the image has appeared behind a distant object, partially obscuring it, such as a window. In these instances, the size of the object and its distance from the camera could be accurately determined.

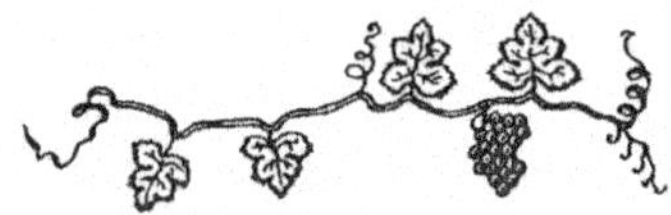

My room at the Buddhist centre in Carlton North remains an important part of the history of SP experiences in my life because I underwent a very large number of SP episodes during the three years I stayed there. Did this have something to do with its location, I wonder? Is the frequency or intensity of SP episodes in any way related to location? It would appear that the answer is yes. Studies have revealed a possible link between the prevalence of SP episodes and fluctuations in geomagnetic activity, a theory I'll explore in a later chapter.

Whenever I sleep at a new location for the first time – such as the house of a relative or friend, or a motel room – the "local" spirits will often take an interest in my being there and will make me aware of their presence, as if to let me know that I've entered their "territory." They might tap me lightly on the shoulder, or grasp me by the hand, as though attempting to shake it. Such actions are quite harmless, if not a little annoying. There have been occasions, however, when my presence was clearly not welcome. On those occasions, I might be attacked quite violently – the strangling I endured is a typical example. Or I might be pushed around and shoved forcefully.

I remember very clearly an incident that occurred several years ago when I slept over for the first time at my sister's place in Healesville. She had recently moved down from Rockhampton, Queensland, and had been renting the house for about five months. Being the home of not just my sister but also her four young children, the house was a crowded, noisy place.

For most of the night I slept rather lightly. I remember waking up once to go to the bathroom. Sometime after midnight, while I was dreaming, I became aware of a presence nearby. My attention was drawn away from my dream, and I then found myself in a mild SP state. At that point, the presence was very strong; I could smell two souls in the room, and they didn't seem particularly friendly, nor, for that matter, did they seem especially mean. They were gruff and insensitive more than anything else and seemed to belong to the elemental category. Using considerable force, they grabbed me by the hands, one on each side, and attempted to drag me out of bed. I woke up properly a couple of seconds later. From what I could gather, they found my presence threatening and did not like my staying in the house, so had decided to do something about it – bouncer style.

There's one elemental that's been with me for many years now. I've named him Arnold. It's an absurd name, I know, but it seems to suit him perfectly. Although I use the word "him," Arnold doesn't seem to be either male or female; he is, to the best of my knowledge, androgynous. Whenever I encounter Arnold – during the SP state, that is – he appears to be attached to my body in some fashion, much in the same way that cleaner fish are "attached" to much larger fish, so as to feed off the dead skin and parasites on their bodies.

Embarrassing though it sounds, Arnold will often lie close to my body, as though trying to soak up some warmth and affection. He will sometimes wake me up several times in the one night, either by shifting positions in bed or by putting his arms around my body. His actions might sound rather sexual, but, I assure you, they're not. What he craves is contact – nothing more. In many ways he reminds me of a cuddly child.

On those nights that I do encounter Arnold, I will usually become aware of his presence at least three or four times. And, as I said, he will often unintentionally wake me up. What seems to be happening is that I somehow remain in a very light SP state for the whole night – or most of the night. It is, it seems, only during these very rare and unusual states of SP that Arnold is able to make his presence known. Unlike many of the beings I encounter and have encountered during SP episodes, Arnold is absolutely harmless.

The SP episodes I experience when he "visits" differ from the norm. They are more external than internal, in the sense that Arnold does not try to enter my mind or take possession of my body. There is less in the way of mind-to-mind contact and more in the way of sensation. I am able to feel Arnold's body next to mine just as if I were lying next to a living person. I can felt the rise and fall of his chest as he breathes in and out. I even feel the beating of his heart.

I mentioned earlier that my room in Carlton North was a place of particularly high SP activity. That this may have been due to the presence of a large number of spirits in the general vicinity, or maybe in my bedroom alone, is one possibility worth considering. After all, before it was transformed into a Buddhist centre, the place was a nursing home. Back then, many elderly people would have lived there, suffered there, and presumably died there.

Another factor worth taking into account is the Buddhist center's close proximity to the Melbourne cemetery. One does wonder, however, whether spirits would actually want to hang out at a cemetery, which is obviously not a place where people die (I have yet to come across a story of someone dropping dead at a funeral service, but I'm sure it's happened), but a place where the bodies of the dead are ceremonially interred. If I were the spirit of a recently deceased person, I'm sure I could think of a much better place to hang out than a dreary cemetery.

But according to that famous book of the Spiritists, *The Spirits' Book* (1856), the idea of spirits "haunting" a graveyard is not as ridiculous as it sounds. On the day of their funerals, it explains, "spirits go to cemeteries in great numbers… called thither by the thoughts of a greater number of persons, but each spirit goes solely for his own friends, and not for the crowd of those who care nothing about him." In *The Mediums' Book* (1861), another Spiritist work, we are told that spirits, "may, for a time, retain a preference for certain places; but those who do so are spirits of inferior advancement." We will return to these books later on, as they both contain valuable information on the nature of invisible, incorporeal beings – information that, in my experience, checks out completely.

CHAPTER 3

A Search For Answers

In 2007, when I wasn't working as a builder's assistant or doing my one class a week at RMIT University, I would be sitting at my desk, typing away on the computer. I wrote a lot of articles that year. When I was stuck for article ideas, I would often scan the internet news websites for inspiration. In April or May, I came across a compelling article on the Science News Online website, called "Night of the Crusher," by Bruce Bower. What immediately caught my interest was the article's subheading: "The waking nightmare of sleep paralysis propels people into a spirit world."

Having read the article, I was much relieved to discover that a label existed for my strange, nocturnal experiences. It was comforting to realize that other people had also had such experiences and knew exactly how I felt. At the same time, however, I found it disquieting to think that the SP phenomenon was so prevalent. If, I asked myself at the time, incorporeal beings are responsible for SP attacks, does this mean they populate our surroundings, and that some of them wish to cause us harm? The answer to both of these questions, I now realize, is most certainly yes.

Bower's article gives a good overview of the SP phenomenon but makes the mistake of implying that these experiences have a physiological basis and nothing more. The possibility that SP experiences could be caused by something of a paranormal nature is totally ignored. Bower seems to believe that the SP phenomenon is partially responsible for mankind's belief in spirits and other "supernatural" beings, and that this phenomenon helped create such "superstitions." Almost every scientist who has studied the SP phenomenon shares this same narrow perspective.

Bower explains that there appears to be a connection between SP, post-traumatic stress disorder (PTSD), and panic attacks, as shown by a number of studies, such as one carried out, in 2003, by psychiatrist Devon E. Hinton of Lowell, Massachusetts, involving 100 of his patients, all of them Cambodian refugees. (Lowell has the second-largest Cambodian population in America.) Forty-two of the 100 patients questioned reported having at least one SP episode each year. In total, 45 of his patients had been diagnosed with PTSD. Of those, 35 reported being afflicted by sleep paralysis, usually with at least one episode a month.

Apparently, SP attacks are traditionally known among Cambodians as "the ghost pushes you down" and that the spirits of the dead cause these attacks. "The Cambodians told Hinton that sleep paralysis permits people who suffer unjust deaths to haunt the living and creates 'bad luck,'" writes Bower. Most of the attacks Hinton's patients described involved seeing demons or other entities and feeling a pressure on the chest.

Given the fact that the subjects used in Hinton's study were all Cambodian refugees, many of them had undergone traumatic events in their lives and therefore suffered from PTSD and other mental disorders. One of Hinton's patients, a woman in her late-forties, had been living in Cambodia during the reign of Pol Pot and had heard three of her friends being clubbed to death by a group of soldiers. An SP sufferer, the woman would often wake up paralyzed and find herself surrounded by "demons with long fangs." These frightening beings, she believed, were the spirits of her executed friends come back to haunt her.

Hinton found that many Cambodian refugees relived traumatic events from their past through their SP experiences, as the case with this woman who suffered from PTSD. According to Hinton, his patients' cultural beliefs in the supernatural – one of them being that the spirits of the dead are able to haunt the living and cause bad luck – were responsible for fostering panic attacks, which in turn were responsible for bringing about SP episodes. A vicious cycle, it seems. Bower gives a summary of Hinton's findings: "Panic attacks, PTSD, and other mental disorders may indirectly promote sleep paralysis by disrupting the sleep cycle and yanking people out of REM sleep during the night...Other factors that disturb sleep, such as jet lag and shift work, have also been linked to sleep paralysis."

In Hinton's opinion, SP episodes are purely psychological and physiological occurrences; they have nothing to do with the paranormal. He believes that simply by placing a paranormal label on these experiences and saying they're caused by spirits and demons creates anxiety for the SP sufferer, which feeds their SP episodes. Sensible though this view is, there's one crucial factor that Hinton's failed to take into account – most SP sufferers are always going to believe that their experiences have a paranormal cause. To deny otherwise would require one to lie to oneself. It's the same as if one day I encountered an alien while walking alone in the forest, communicated with him telepathically for hours, took a ride in his flying saucer, but later decided that I must have been deluding myself, and that the so called alien I'd met was probably just a kid with an abnormally large head. A ridiculous example, no doubt, but I'm sure the reader can grasp my point.

When I began to research the SP phenomenon in early 2007, I quickly realized that there was scant information available about it, especially in book form. I managed to track down a number of interesting articles about SP on the internet, but that's about it. Drawing from what little information I could find, as well as my own personal experiences, I decided to write an article on the subject, which was later published in *New Dawn* magazine, under the title "Mind Parasites and the World of Invisible Spirits."

That my article was written from the perspective of someone who believes in the paranormal, and, more importantly, from someone who has experienced the SP phenomenon first-hand, was very significant, I thought, because most of material I had come across on the topic had been written by narrow-minded skeptics who had never experienced the phenomenon themselves. One cannot begin to understand the SP phenomenon without having had a single SP episode – or, more accurately, without having had numerous SP episodes, and of various kinds. Obviously, each episode is different, varying, for example, from a short bout of paralysis to a full blown OBE accompanied by malicious entities.

Because I wished to include details of my own SP experiences in my "Mind Parasites" article, yet did not want to jeopardize my reputation, I decided to give myself the pseudonym "Joe" and make him an interviewee. This allowed me to describe my experiences as honestly and intimately as I liked, without embarrassing myself, and without giving my readers the impression that I was stark-raving mad.

Not long after the article was published, I received several emails from readers who described having experiences similar to "Joe's." One was from a woman who obviously suffered from a serious mental illness and was clearly very disturbed and unhappy. I will call her Mary. Each email she sent me was more bizarre than the last. She claimed that several creatures – which she called "critters" – had invaded her "aura" and would keep her up at night by buzzing loudly. Apparently, they would speak to her. By far the strangest thing she said is that the "critters" would place insects in her mouth at night. When she would eventually spit them out, in large quantities, a sticky substance accompanied them.

She had placed some of the insects, still encompassed in globules of her own saliva, into small, plastic containers, which she had then put in the freezer. She sent me photographs of these "frozen spit insects," which looked like nothing more than gnats and such. She even sent me photographs of her dried mucus that contained insects. Naturally, my reaction was one of nausea. I disposed of the photographs immediately.

Although many of Mary's claims were difficult to take seriously and seemed like nothing more than the paranoid delusions of a schizophrenic, I sensed that her story contained a grain of truth. She was not an SP sufferer in the normal sense – that was clear – although, curiously, some of her "critter" encounters featured elements of SP attacks, including those experiences that took place while she was fully awake. The thought occurred to me that she may have been a victim of spirit possession. Not wanting to feed her possible delusions, however, I kept this to myself and eventually decided to cease corresponding with her.

Mary wrote me a poignant account of how the "critters" became a part of her life. Born in Poland, Mary and her family were forced to flee the country at the end of World War II and ended up migrating to Germany. Many of her family members died as a result of the war, including her father. She felt depressed and alone in Germany, and not at all at home. A year after getting married, Mary and her husband migrated to Australia and had two children. "Life was good," she says, "[it] had its ups and downs and it did pass very quickly." Tragically, the day before they were planning to move to Queensland to retire, Mary's husband died of a heart attack, so she went there alone. It was then that she started to have disturbing paranormal experiences and became aware of an unwelcome, non-physical presence. "I had the feeling that I was not on my own."

Getting to sleep at night became difficult, as Mary was frequently bothered by a buzzing noise, which she initially attributed to mosquitoes and other insects. Using insect spray had no effect, however. Sometimes, too, she felt as though "something was running up and down [inside] the mattress." Thinking that mice might be responsible, she set up numerous traps but caught nothing. Shortly afterwards, Mary saw, for a fraction of a second, an entity with the appearance of a jellyfish. It jumped out of her bed, she says, just after she had replaced the doona. Although the creature moved with the speed of a mouse, quickly disappearing under the bed, Mary managed to get a clear look at it. It was about the size of her hand, light orange in color, and "had very fine black stripes," as though they'd been "painted on by an artist."

Mary went to the doctor, was diagnosed as mentally ill (most likely schizophrenic), and was prescribed some kind of medication, presumably of the antipsychotic variety. (These details were not included in her account, and I felt it was impolite to obtain them from her.) However, taking the medication did not put an end to her "hallucinations." Visits to psychics and alternative healers to have her aura "cleaned" and such were also of no benefit.

At night, the disturbances continued – and still do to this day. When she goes to bed, Mary often hears, in addition to the loud buzzing sound (sometimes described as a "humming"), a chirping noise, and sometimes breathing, too. "The sound of insects is often very strong, as if the whole room is filled with them." It initially took Mary many hours to get to sleep. Some nights she'd wake up frequently *"from getting so much vibration like electricity through my body"* (my emphasis). Mary came to believe – and still believes – that there are several "critters" living in her aura. Sometimes, while lying in bed, she'll hear them "hopping" on the mattress and will feel their presence beside her, touching her body and breathing in her face. The entities have apparently told Mary that they've been with her since childhood and mean her no harm, though she doesn't trust what they say.

It's not uncommon for SP sufferers to feel and hear what they think is a person breathing in their face. I have experienced this myself. As for the presence in bed, lying beside you, this is quite common. So too is the feeling of vibration. In Mary's case, however, these "hallucinations" are experienced not only while she's in an altered state of consciousness – possibly the SP state – but also while she's fully awake. It would seem that Mary's "critters" are similar in nature to poltergeist entities in that they're allegedly able to produce physical phenomena, such as the placing of insects in her mouth. This occurs while she is "asleep," she says. "I can feel that something is put in my mouth, because my lips always open a bit on the end and I try to keep them very hard closed."

One time, while sitting in the lounge room reading the paper, four little insects mysteriously dropped onto the page, almost as though they'd materialized in the air above her. On another occasion, also while reading, Mary felt something bite her on the arm, "but there was nothing around." She inspected her arm and noticed the presence of blood. According to Mary, the invisible "critters" often bite her on the back of the neck as well, "and that is when I start to feel foggy or I have a veil over my eyes." At times, objects in her house mysteriously disappear, reappearing later in odd locations.

Once again, the accuracy of Mary's story is difficult to determine, and, instead of being wholly real or wholly imaginary, is probably a combination of both. The possibility exists that the traumatic death of her husband rendered her vulnerable to possession by parasitic discarnate entities – similar in nature, perhaps, to the ones I've encountered during SP attacks – which have since being living in, and feeding off, her aura. I will deal with the topic of spirit possession – specifically in regards to SP attacks, poltergeist disturbances, and mental illness – later on.

Also in response to my article, I received, on August 29, 2007, a fascinating email from a female SP sufferer. It was because of this email that I became aware of the close connection that exists between the SP phenomenon and OBEs – a connection I was almost entirely ignorant of when I wrote my "Mind Parasites" article. Here is the text of her email in slightly truncated form, with the woman's name omitted so as to protect her identity:

"Thank you for your article in *New Dawn*. It clarified an incident that happened to me many years ago. I had suffered from quite a few episodes of SP on waking up and I found them very irritating. At first I would try desperately to move but I would inevitably have to wait until the episode passed and I fully woke up. However I can recall a particular incident which to this day has amazed me, as I don't really know what happened.

"At this point I suppose I should clarify that I was not and am not on any medication and I have not suffered metal illness of any kind. I teach Chemistry and Mathematics and value reason, logic and proof but I am also open-minded and intrigued by the paranormal.

"When I was a young mother about twenty years ago I was taking an afternoon nap while my son was sleeping in the next room. I half woke up with my eyes open but totally paralyzed and I could hear my son crying in the next room. I was desperate to wake up and go and comfort him, and frantically tried to make myself move. Our en suite was opposite my bed so I thought if I could make it over there I could throw some water on my face and I would wake up properly. I made an enormous effort, willing myself to move but popped out of my body and started travelling upwards instead of across the bed to the en suite. Furthermore, I recall there was a slight whooshing sound as I travelled upwards and out of my body. I quickly panicked as I thought I was dead. I started thinking that my son would be left crying in his bed and my husband would come home and find me dead. When I really panicked I returned to my body and instantly woke up.

"For the past 10 years I have not suffered at all from SP. There are a few memories prior to this incident. As a child I remember waking up at night and feeling certain I was not in my bed but level with the light on the ceiling. I reached up and touched the ceiling to prove it to myself. I dismissed it as a dream and didn't think about it until years later. Also you mention

'Joe' hearing voices. I recall one afternoon sleep when I woke with SP and I heard female voices whispering next to my bed, but couldn't see anyone and I was definitely the only person in the house at the time. I remember sensing (and this could be rubbish) that it was my dead grandma talking about me.

"Although simple, these incidents, as in Joe's case, have affected me spiritually. Anyway when I read your article it brought back memories..."

Luckily for the SP sufferer (and perhaps, in some cases, unluckily), little effort is needed to have an OBE because the SP state is highly conducive to such experiences. It is a doorway into the realm of the paranormal. Like the shaman, chronic SP sufferers have a foot in both worlds. They have access to a whole other reality that few people realize exists.

Since beginning work on this book, I've discussed the subject of SP with numerous friends and acquaintances, and have found that those most likely to be directly familiar with the phenomenon – and to have had, for example, at least a few compelling SP experiences – are generally individuals who have an active dream life and who seem to possess at least some degree of psychic ability. (It should be mentioned, however, that many of these individuals had not heard of the term sleep paralysis and did not know it to be a sleep condition prior to my having informed them about it.)

I was not at all surprised when one such friend of mine, the conspiracy author Aeolus Kephas – an experienced lucid dreamer – revealed, during an online radio show, that he had had encounters with "inorganic beings" – what were also referred to as "angels" and "demons" – and that these encounters had taken place during the SP state. Author of *The Lucid View: Investigations Into Occultism, Ufology and Paranoid Awareness*, Kephas is a deep thinker and a man of considerable intellect whose writings demonstrate a profound understanding of magick and occultism – what he calls sorcery. Kephas considers himself a sorcerer of sorts and is certainly no stranger to altered states of consciousness and mysterious experiences in general.

Kephas was generous enough to send me a detailed account of his SP experiences. The following was written in early 2009, long after I'd completed the second draft of this book, which, by the way, Kephas did not read and knew very little about. His experiences and observations are extremely similar to my own.

"My experiences of sleep paralysis have almost always entailed the irrefutable certainty of a non-human presence in the room," wrote Kephas.

"Since I was never under the impression of there being a fully physical or even visible presence, however, the presence might best be described as a conscious energy field. Not that I ever opened my eyes to look; that was never an option. My bodily reaction to the presence was invariably one of terror and, as such, the last thing I intended to do was try and see the being. It was quite overwhelming enough merely to experience its energy field as a form of 'psychic sensation.' I don't know how else to describe it. I was aware of a consciousness outside of my own, immeasurably more powerful, and focused on me in such a way that it was akin to a kind of psychic assault or 'ambush.' The being or presence was not hostile; far from it. It seemed to be interested in me not in any predatory manner but rather almost in a propriety way, almost as with the attention of a lover, or perhaps a loving but ruthless parent?

"As I recall I had a series of very similar experiences – I might say "visitations" –during a period of a couple of years when I was in my late 20s. Since I was quite deeply influenced by [Whitley] Strieber's *Communion* at that time, I tended to see my experiences in the light of Strieber's own accounts, and this may have influenced or even distorted my impressions somewhat. I definitely had a sense that the being—if such it was—was 'ancient,' wise, and extremely powerful, and essentially benevolent. On at least a couple of occasions, I experienced it as female (I knew nothing of the Old Hag syndrome back then). And although it sounds rather fanciful now, I had a sense more than once that it, she, was 'my own soul,' or as close as made no difference. Anima visitation?

"The experience of paralysis was an intrinsic part of the visitation. Each time, while in the process of falling asleep, in that precise moment in which the conscious mind recedes and dreaming begins, I entered into an alternate state in which my mind was fully awake and yet my body seemed to be totally asleep, paralyzed. This realization was simultaneous with a far more shocking awareness of an "alien energy field" having "arrived" in the bedroom, as if from nowhere. So it was as if, in that moment of slipping from one state to the next (as the assemblage point began to move?), a crack between worlds appeared and some entity had managed to materialize, in my room, as a physical presence.

"There was nothing subjective or vague about the experience; at the time there was no more doubt in my mind that something very real was present than there would be if a burglar had come through the window, wielding a crowbar. Yet as I say, there was nothing visual about the experience, nor was there any sound, smell, or even an ordinary sensation to speak of (i.e., of being touched). Whatever senses were alerted related to consciousness itself, not to the ordinary five bodily senses. And yet, it was above all a bodily sensation that alerted me—what Strieber called 'body terror.' Rather than an awareness of the presence causing the terror, however, it was as if my own terror informed me as to the being's presence. Somehow, my body knew instantly that some unknown form of energy was present, and it reacted with a kind of animal terror. My mind, on the other hand, observed this physiological response with a measure of detachment and, of course, of fascination. I felt something like love emanating from the being, and even felt something similar in myself responding to that love. But there was a seemingly unbridgeable abyss between us – that of our individual physical or energetic configurations. We were quite literally worlds apart."

Kepahs then went on to describe another, less positive form of sleep paralysis visitation: "I suffered a recurring dream over the years. There was something on my back, clinging to me. I could feel it like an electrical charge, like something actually drilling into the back of my neck. I could hear a strange voice or voices, and knew that some 'being' was working on me. In order to stop it, I shrugged my shoulders physically, once, twice, a third time, until my consciousness returned to my body and I woke. I had the feeling the being was still there, however, waiting for a second chance to 'leech' me.

"It was like a child suckling, a small but ferocious creature. Whatever it was, it was clinging to me with desperate persistence, chewing at my neck, drinking my energy like a vampire. At the time, it felt like a physical thing. If I was in 'the astral' at the time, then I suppose it was as solid as I was. Even at the time, however, I could hardly believe what I was feeling. A horrible, nightmarish parasite entity feeding off me, relentlessly and without mercy, maybe even without choice? It was like a part of me. It had been attracted by my energy, we were like two magnets. The effect was of repulsion more than terror. This demon was something utterly and undeniably real. The source of all my sickness was here.

"How vile to share one's life force with some mindless, soulless succubus! Now it was finally clear, beyond any doubt. My Soul was trapped, caught in the snares of some dark and malevolent force, like a fly in a web."

CHAPTER 4

The Terror That Comes In The Night

One of the great pioneers of SP research is David J. Hufford, University Professor Emeritus of Medical Humanities at PennState College of Medicine and Adjunct Professor of Religious Studies at the University of Pennsylvania, and author of *The Terror That Comes in the Night*. In 1964, while a university student, Hufford had an SP experience of his own. It was nearing the end of the year, and Hufford, sick with mononucleosis, had been busy studying for his finals. Feeling exhausted, he decided to take a nap in his room. He soon drifted into a deep sleep but woke up an hour later to the sound of the bedroom door creaking open, which he had locked securely before going to bed. He then heard the sound of approaching footsteps – a common feature of the SP phenomenon. There was, he thought, an evil presence in the room.

Unable to move a muscle but with his eyes open, Hufford became increasingly frightened with each passing moment. He felt a heavy weight on his chest as the "malevolent entity" jumped on top of him. It put its ghostly hands around his neck and began to squeeze. As he struggled to breathe, Hufford thought he was going to die. At that moment, however, the SP attack suddenly ended, and, able to move once more, Hufford jumped out of bed and ran out of the room, taking refuge in the student union.

It wasn't until 1971, when he moved to Newfoundland, that Hufford encountered the SP phenomenon again – this time as a researcher. What was once known as Newfoundland is now called Newfoundland and Labrador. Labrador is a region of mainland Canada. It and the island of Newfoundland, separated by the Strait of Belle Isle, form one province. Newfoundland has been compared in size to the state of Pennsylvania in the U.S., with an area of about 108,860 square kilometers. Hufford mentions that because of its geographical and historical isolation, Newfoundland is culturally "distinct and fascinating."

During the three years that he called Newfoundland home, Hufford worked as a faculty member in the Folklore Department of Memorial University, located in the capitol St. John's. As part of his work there, Hufford was given various archival duties. The people of the island, he discovered, were no strangers to the realm of the paranormal, as evidenced by the fact that the archives contained a large quantity of folk belief material pertaining to a wide variety of topics, including fairies, ghost ships, Will-o'-the-Wisps, and many others. It wasn't long before he came across the Old Hag tradition, of which most people in the island were familiar. A twenty-year-old, university student living on the island defined the experience as follows: "You are dreaming and you feel as if someone is holding you down. You can do nothing, only cry out. People believe that you will die if you are not awakened."

Although commonly known as "the Old Hag," the SP phenomenon, Hufford discovered, was known by many other names as well, such as the "diddies," "the hags," and "hag rid." To have had such an experience was to have been "hagged." The term "the Old Hag" was also used to refer to the person or supernatural entity believed to be responsible for the attack. According to the Old Hag tradition, these attacks are not only caused by evil spirits and demons but by humans as well, and sometimes a combination of the two. It might be that the "hag," or evil spirit, has acted independently, or has been called on by a witch or a sorcerer to carry out the attack. It is also believed that witches and so on, having the ability to temporarily leave their physical bodies, can operate as a spirit and "hag" their victims that way.

Included in Hufford's book is an interview with an eighty-year-old native of Newfoundland whose story reveals a lot about the Old Hag phenomenon and its relationship to witchcraft. The man was thirty at the time and had been working in Labrador, supposedly as a fisherman. One night, while staying in a bunkhouse, he and the other men met an attractive young woman, "a bedroom a girl," whom his friend tried unsuccessfully to seduce. His friend threatened the girl, saying he'd "hag" her in the night if she didn't let him kiss her. But the girl took no notice of the warning. "Anyway he went home and...that was the night he hagged her! and hagged her good."

It was after the girl had gone home to bed that the man's friend began "hagging" her. As part of the ritual he conducted, the man removed his clothes and knelt beside the bed. "I was there watchin' him when he done it...He said the Lord's Prayer backwards; then jumped under the covers and took a knife from under the pilla and stuck it in the sideboard three or four times...Every now and then we'd hear him bawl out, 'Hag, good Hag!' And that's how he hagged her." Apparently, while the girl was being "hagged," she could see her attacker "standin' over her with the knife; and she couldn't move because she was stopped still with fright. The foam was even comin' out of her mouth, and her father only got her back to sense by callin' her name backwards." The man adds: "His spirit...was what hagged her."

Although this anecdote sounds completely farfetched, there is, I think, a ring of truth to it. In this case, what brought about the girl's ghastly SP episode was a kind of "psychic attack." Angered by the fact that he could not "possess" the girl's body, the man decided to take his revenge on her and prove his dominance by attacking her in spirit form. That this anecdote has strong sexual overtones cannot be denied. I explained earlier that an SP attack could be likened to a kind of rape, and this case seems to support that view.

According to the British occultist Dion Fortune in her classic book *Psychic Self-Defence*, when an occultist wishes to attack someone psychically they usually wait until their victim is asleep, because that is when one is most vulnerable to psychic influences. The reason for this is quite logical when one considers the fact that while we're asleep the conscious mind has retired for the day, leaving the unconscious mind in charge. One's "psychic guard" is down at this time, so to speak. The man who "hagged" the young woman must have known this.

Included in Hufford's book is another account of an Old Hag attack that seems to be related to witchcraft. A sixty-year-old woman, whose name is not given, told the story to two of Hufford's students. The case took place in 1915 and involved three people between eighteen and twenty years of age: a Salvation Army schoolteacher named Robert, a workman named John, and his girlfriend, Jean. Robert fancied Jean and attempted to steal her from John. About a month later, "Robert began to be hagged. Every night when he went to bed, it was as if someone was pressing across his chest – it was as if he we was being strangled. Robert became so sick that the people he boarded with thought he was going to die."

So as to defeat the "hag," Robert went to bed one night with a board placed across his chest and a pocketknife held between his hands, the blade retracted. "It was hoped that when the hag came to lie across his chest, the hag would be killed." The following morning, Robert woke up to find the pocketknife embedded in the piece of board. "Only for the board Robert would have been killed...Robert knew that John...was the person who was hagging him. He put it down to jealousy on John's part...*The hag was brought about by a curse*" (my emphasis).

It's difficult to know what to make of this case. Some of the details are obviously nonsense, especially the part about the pocketknife being embedded in the piece of wood. Clearly, Robert thought his nocturnal attacker – the "hag" – was a physical being, and thus attempted to defeat it using physical means. In comparison to the previous case, in which the man's spirit was said to have caused the attack, this case, it seems, involved something else – something acting independently of John, the supposed attacker. It's as though John had felt such anger towards Robert that he put a curse on him, either consciously or unconsciously, which attracted the assistance of an evil spirit. Or at least that's one interpretation.

When an occultist or shaman wishes to place a curse on someone, he is, as a general rule, unable to succeed independently and must employ the assistance of evil spirits (or an evil spirit), for they are able to act on a level that he is not. Being inhabitants of the astral realm, they operate on an astral level; it is their natural habitat, and this makes them masters of that realm. One could say that fish and other aquatic animals are masters of the environment they inhabit – the ocean – and that man is master of the environment he inhabits – dry land. Although man possesses a dimension of mind that operates on an astral level, our natural environment is the physical, material world. In our present state as physical beings, the nature of the astral realm is beyond our ability to fully comprehend or manipulate.

The evil spirits that sorcerers employ to do their bidding operate as intermediaries between them and their victims. To explain this better, I feel it necessary to provide the reader with an accurate definition of the word "intermediary," as given by the *Penguin English Dictionary*: "Somebody or something acting as a mediator or go between." Because psychic attacks occur on an immaterial, or astral, level, it is necessary for the sorcerer to employ the use of an intermediary – i.e. spirit – to help him effect change on that level.

During the course of his research, Hufford interviewed a great many number of SP suffers, not all of them from Newfoundland and not all of them university students. Some of them were unfamiliar with the Old Hag tradition and had never heard of such experiences. They were, in other words, completely ignorant of the phenomenon, so there was no possibility that their cultural background was responsible for coloring, or creating, their experiences. One such person – "who stated ignorance of both the tradition and the experiences of others" – was a man in his mid-thirties named John who worked as an executive at the time the interview was conducted. "The [SP] victim is frequently someone who, like John, disclaims any general belief or interest in the supernatural and insists that he has never had any other unusual experiences," writes Hufford.

At age fifteen, while staying with his grandparent's in their two-storey house, John had a series of frightening SP experiences, which occurred five nights in a row. The room in which he was staying permitted a view of the stairway. On the first night, while lying in bed, he heard footsteps coming up the stairs. John was unable to move or cry out, but was able to open and close his eyes and gaze around the room. He saw a figure come up the stairway, walk down the hallway, and enter his room. "And it was almost all white and glowing. It had a hat on. It was dressed like an elderly lady." The figure sat down on the floor, "and it looked to me like an elephant of all things. Just a blob, but white...And I broke out into a sweat and was just forced onto the bed." Describing what he saw in greater detail, John said the old woman was transformed into a white blob, and that this blob had "the general impression of an elephant."

Thinking it would sound "ridiculous," John did not mention the incident to anyone. But he did ask his grandmother about the mysterious footsteps, explaining that he thought he heard someone coming up the stairs late at night. This noise, she said, was probably caused by the linoleum floor, which, after getting pushed down during the day, tends to rise up at night. But this made no sense to John: "these were definite footsteps..." The next night, while sleeping in the same room, this time accompanied by his grandmother who was there to comfort him, the same experience occurred again. He heard, once more, the sound of approaching footsteps; then he saw the white blob.

John stayed in the house three more nights, and on each of those nights the mysterious "white blob" made an appearance. Although he heard the entity and was aware of its presence in the room, he was too frightened to open his eyes. He therefore saw the being on only two occasions. That he underwent the experience five nights in a row is quite startling, as this is rare among SP sufferers, but certainly not unheard of.

A young woman named Caroline provided Hufford with an equally frightening personal account of an SP attack. A graduate student from the U.S., she had been living in Newfoundland for only a few months at the time her experience occurred. Caroline described waking up in the night – "or I thought I woke up" – and finding herself in a state of paralysis, unable to make a sound. She was, she said, conscious of her surroundings and able to look around her room. There appeared to be a man lying next to her, holding her arm. His head was resting on her shoulder. She thought the "man" was asleep, and was greatly disturbed by his presence. "And then I tried to scream. But I couldn't get any sound out." Each time she tried to move, so as to get a glimpse of the "man's" face, she felt her arm being gripped tighter. The "man" kept moving closer towards her. "And I started thinking, 'Now if I move again, he's going to rape me.'"

The "man," she said, had a very strong odor, "all sweaty and kind of dusty." (According to Hufford, SP sufferers very rarely report gustatory hallucinations.) The next thing she knew, the "man" was lying on top of her. Able to move her neck ever so slightly, she managed to catch a glimpse of his head. He appeared to be wearing "a really funny, ghastly-looking kind of mask." Before long, the SP attack came to an end, and the "masked man" disappeared. Caroline told Hufford that she "was conscious of seeing the whole room," though it was "kind of hazy...It wasn't real clear but it wasn't like a dream either." Some people, myself included, are able to see their surroundings quite clearly during SP experiences.

The Terror That Comes in the Night describes a few other cases in which the SP sufferer was able to get a clear look at his or her attacker while the episode was underway. Humanlike attackers are more commonly seen than non-human attackers, says Hufford. "In all visual cases," he adds, "whether the attacker is humanlike, animal, or something else, the detail most frequently commented on is the eyes." Interestingly, in cases of alien abduction, abductees often describe the eyes of these entities as being of great significance. In *Passport to the Cosmos*, John E. Mack's final book on the close encounter phenomenon, he writes: "The large eyes of the beings are consistently reported to be by far the most prominent feature of their faces, and an important locus of connection."

Included in Hufford's book is an interview with a man in his early twenties named Ron, who during his senior year of college had a terrifying encounter with an evil "murky presence" with "a glaring stare to it." Feeling "dead tired," Ron decided to take an afternoon nap. He soon drifted into a very deep sleep, but was suddenly woken up by the sound of the door slamming. Although unable to move, Ron managed to open his eyes, and was able to see quite clearly. He noticed the door was still closed, and that his roommate had not entered the room as suspected. Ron felt a great pressure on his body, which gradually increased in intensity. "And the next thing I knew I was, like, totally wiped out. I just lay there."

Glancing at the clock beside his bed, Ron took note of the time. He then saw a "grayish, brownish murky presence" sweep towards him from a darkened area of the room, changing from a gaseous blob into a rectangular-shaped creature with sharp edges. It approached the bed "and kind of stood over me with a glare." That the entity seemed to be glaring struck

Ron as very strange because it "had no real face...For some reason, I got a feeling of a real cold stare from it..." Ron very definitely felt menace emanating from the entity. "This was evil! You know, this is weird!" As the being began to "envelope the bed," the pressure was so intense that Ron felt as though he were being crushed to death.

As Ron struggled in terror to free himself, he could hear various noises in the background – normal noises – of stereos playing and people doing things in the rooms adjoining his. He felt, at the time, as though he were fully awake. Before long, the experience "kind of dissipated away. The presence, everything." Checking the time once more, Ron noticed that five minutes had elapsed. Even though his mind had shifted from an altered state of consciousness to a fully awake state of consciousness, the background noises continued as normal. This seems to indicate that Ron's experience had little in common with a dream. It turns out that nobody had entered the room while he was asleep. Nor had anybody slammed the door or heard it slam. (A door slamming sound is commonly reported by SP sufferers but not as often as the sound of footsteps.)

Another individual Hufford interviewed, a twenty-three-year-old medical student named Jack, described seeing a seven-foot-tall, caped and silhouetted figure with "very dark eyes." As he lay on his bed in a state of fear and paralysis, Jack couldn't help but stare at the figure. It had long brown hair and appeared to be wearing a hat of some sort. But the detail that caught Jack's attention the most was the entity's "very piercing eyes. They were just looking at me...They were eyes and it sent a chill up my spine – tingling, you know, shivering type of sensation."

Jack's first SP experiences occurred when he was in his early teens, when he and his brother were required to share the same bed. There were times, says Jack, in which his brother would be awake while he was having an attack. Jack's brother would notice that Jack's eyes were open, "just staring straight out into space," and that his breathing sounded heavy and unusual. During these occasions, Jack's brother noticed nothing of a paranormal nature. He did not see, for instance, a hooded figure standing near the bed, staring at Jack. This seems to be true of most SP cases in which a second party is present at the time of the disturbance.

Ron had had a similar experience: he thought he'd heard the sound of a slamming door – a sound so loud it apparently woke him up – but later learned that no one else had heard any such thing. It would be easy to conclude that the sound existed only in Ron's head and was therefore a purely subjective experience – an explanation I find inadequate. The late Michael

Talbot, author of *The Holographic Universe*, came up with the term "omnijective" to explain the nature of certain types of paranormal phenomena, particularly UFOs. The term is used to refer to something that is neither objective nor subjective, but halfway in-between. This, I think, is the best way to classify the hallucinations of SP sufferers.

The sound Ron heard was a psychic impression – an "astral sound," so to speak – and it's quite possible that had someone else been with him at the time, and in the same receptive state of consciousness, they too would have heard it or perhaps something like it. It should be borne in mind, however, that psychic impressions are never totally "clean," in the sense that one's conscious mind colors the information received by the intuitive unconscious mind. This phenomenon is well-recognized by parapsychologists, and in the field of remote viewing it's called "analytical overlay" (AOL).

It would appear that the mind of the SP sufferer plays a role in giving shape to the entities you see. Support for this theory can be found in the accounts given by Ron and John respectively. In John's case, the being he saw transformed from an old lady into a white blob that resembled an elephant. And in Ron's case, as the murky, gaseous presence approached him from across the room, it morphed into a being with eyes and a rectangular-shaped body. Of course, it's impossible to prove in either of these cases that John and Ron were responsible, partially or otherwise, for the transformation of the beings they saw; perhaps they changed of their own accord.

Most but not all of the SP sufferers Hufford interviewed for his book said they found their experiences frightening. Pat, a young woman from California, told Hufford that, as a child, her bed would sometimes start rocking on its own, "up and down, back and forth." Initially frightened by the mysterious sensation, Pat eventually started to enjoy it. As a young teenager, she would often sense a presence in the room and hear a strange "snurfling" sound. One time she saw an ape-like creature with glowing red eyes.

I too have experienced a rocking bed sensation, although I can't say I found it enjoyable. It feels as if someone is standing at the foot of the bed, pushing it back and forth. Whenever it's happened to me, I've been able to sense an unpleasant presence in the room. The mischievous spirits responsible could hardly be called quitters because the rocking sometimes goes on for what seems like hours. Certain spirits, it seems, have mastered the art of being annoying. Anyone who's had dealings with what *The Spirits' Book* calls "imperfect spirits" will tell you that they're very persistent.

Some of my most terrifying nightmares have all occurred prior to SP episodes, leading me to conclude that spirits are able to influence one's dreams, and do it in a very unpleasant way. Other SP sufferers have reported the same thing. The dreams preceding SP episodes, says Hufford, "tend to be frightening and violent" and are "generally incongruous" in that they don't relate to anything that the dreamer has been thinking about. In my experience, these dreams have all been very strange and foreign, as though they were implanted in my mind, so as to induce a strong emotional reaction of fear and helplessness.

One person who, in Hufford's book, reported having strange dreams prior to an SP episode was a twenty-three-year-old medical student named George. The attack took place on the second floor of the university library, where George had been busy studying for an exam. Feeling exhausted – for he had been getting about four hours sleep a night – George decided to take a quick nap on one of the couches. Lying on his back with his hands across his chest, he soon drifted to sleep. "And I had a series of about three or four very quick dreams, which to me made no sense, because they really didn't pertain to anything that...was familiar to me. They were very obscure episodes...semi-frightening in nature, and also quite violent. One of them had to do with an animal. What kind of animal, I don't know. It was a very strange type of animal. But there was also, you know, 'Why would I conjure up this unusual animal?'"

As he lay there, paralyzed, George heard someone approach from behind. Judging by the sound of their footsteps, it appeared to be a woman wearing heels. George was hoping that she, whoever she was, would walk past him, and not "mess with me." He then heard a female voice that he could not recognize. "But the voice addressed me like she knew me. Or it knew me. And it said, 'You knew that I would come.' Something like that. And then there was a lot of talk about her – her face. Or her appearance. And she didn't want me to look at her or something, because of her face." The woman's voice, said George, was "very calm." That it spoke to him "like it knew me" troubled and confused him.

The voice continued speaking, but George was unable to make out the words. He grew nervous. He then felt two hands press down on his arms. George tried to struggle against the pressure but was unable to move an inch. He also tried to scream, but no sound would come out of his mouth. Having opened his eyes, George saw nothing out of the ordinary. The woman he thought he'd see was simply not there. The attack came to an end when George took a calm and rational approach to what he was experiencing. He successfully moved his left hand, "and soon all the pressure was gone, and I sat up. And there was nothing there…"

George told Hufford that "every time I've slept in the library I've always had unusual dreams." In his conservative way, Hufford suggests that certain locations – such as the library in George's case – "may indicate the presence of an external variable in the causation of the Old Hag attacks." As to what this "external variable" may be, Hufford does not say.

In *The Terror That Comes in the Night*, Hufford devotes a section to the relationship between hauntings and SP attacks, and, although he chooses to remain extremely objective about the matter and draws no conclusions, there can be little doubt that SP victims experience attacks more frequently than usual while sleeping in haunted locations. Of all the cases in Hufford's book that support the "spirit hypothesis," there is one in particular that deserves special mention. Because the haunting occurred in the town of Bowling Green, Kentucky, I have decided to name it "The Ghost of Bowling Green."

PART 2

CHAPTER 5

The Ghost Of Bowling Green

Hufford first heard about the Ghost of Bowling Green case during the spring of 1975, while he was a guest of the Folklore Department at Western Kentucky University. That preceding November, Lynwood Montell, the chairman of the department, had been contacted by two young women, named Carol and Ruth, who claimed that the house they lived in was haunted. Their friend Joan had recently moved out. The disturbances in the house were such that it had become uninhabitable, they declared. Desperate to get help from whomever they could, they had decided to contact the university.

Carol and Ruth provided Montell with a detailed description of the haunting. The interview was recorded, and the tape was then passed on to Hufford. Listening to the tape, Hufford was surprised to discover that all three women gave descriptions of typical Old Hag attacks. His curiosity aroused, he decided to interview the women himself. He managed to locate Carol and Joan, but not Ruth. At the time they had lived in the house together, all three women had been in their early twenties. They had all grown up in Kentucky, and two of them had graduated from Western Kentucky University.

Located out of town, the house was believed to be around one hundred years old. Half of it was of log construction, and it was in this section of the house that Carol's and Joan's bedrooms were located. Unfortunately for Carol and Joan, it also happened to be where most of the disturbances had taken place. For some reason, the spirit occupying the house had been particularly attached to Carol's room. Rumor had it that the previous tenant of the house – a woman – had been involved in witchcraft. But this proved difficult to verify and was later considered to be of no significance to the haunting.

Shortly after they moved into the house on July 15, 1974, all three women began to suffer from nausea and diarrhea, and were diagnosed with hepatitis, due, it was believed, to the consumption of contaminated well water. Two months later, their symptoms inexplicably disappeared, and it was never properly established if hepatitis had indeed been the causes of their illness. The women said that although they sometimes drank alcohol, and occasionally smoked marijuana, this had no bearing on what they experienced while living in the house.

In Hufford's description of the case, he includes excerpts from the transcripts of both interviews – the one conducted by Montell and the one that he conducted. He is quick to point out, moreover, that although his main motivation for speaking to the women was to gain additional details of their Old Hag attacks, he did not let on that this was his purpose, so as not to contaminate the information he was given. He told them, instead, to go over their entire recollection of the haunting. Montell, of course, had spoken to only Carol and Ruth, and Hufford had spoken to only Carol and Joan. "The result was an opportunity to compare the two interviews point by point," writes Hufford, "and I was surprised to find that there were no substantial differences as a result of either time or the addition of a third point of view."

The first strange incident occurred about two weeks after the women had moved in. Ruth, who was alone in the house at the time, fell asleep on the couch in the living room, and began having "a very paranoid dream" in which "everybody was like horribly distorted," and "really cruel-looking." A moment later, Ruth woke up but was unable to move from the couch because "something wouldn't let me!" Right at that moment, Carol and Joan arrived home, waking Ruth up as soon as they entered the living room (presumably unintentionally). The fact that Ruth mentions she was "paralyzed" clearly indicates that what she underwent was an SP attack. So frightening did she find the experience that she became "frantic" and started crying. Despite the fact that it was a very hot day, her body, according to Joan, "was just freezing."

Before long, the women began to hear "strange noises," particularly "thumps," and that of footsteps on the stairs. Sometimes one of the beds would start shaking while nobody was in the room. Most of the sounds came from Carol's upstairs bedroom. According to Ruth and Joan, the ghost tended to be more active while Carol was away at her parent's house. For a while, they were reluctant to tell her about the strange noises in her bedroom, knowing it would only make her feel more frightened than she already was.

One night, while lying in bed, reading, Carol suddenly heard a voice from the air, calling out her name "in a sort of whisper." It was, she said, "a real insistent type tone of voice." Ruth also heard a whispery, disembodied voice. It called out her name two or three times while she was relaxing on the couch. (For some reason, spirits enjoy calling out people's names. This is not only true of hauntings in which the voice is heard while the witness is fully awake, it also occurs frequently in cases of SP. I've heard my name called out numerous times.)

It took some time before the women finally realized that they were not alone in the house. They knew that something was amiss, but they were trying not to give in to their fear. They felt that if they put on a brave face, the problem would eventually disappear. How wrong they were. As time passed, the disturbances in the house increased in frequency and intensity.

The next major event of the haunting occurred after the women decided to paint their old, second-hand refrigerator. Everyone in the house, including some of their friends, had decorated the refrigerator with pictures and messages, and the women were pleased with the results. One of the messages, painted in large letters on the top of the refrigerator, read: "It is the right of the people to throw off such a government." The following day, they discovered to their astonishment that the message had been smeared off, except no one in the house had touched it. The same thing happened again a couple of days later, after the paint had dried; it happened repeatedly, in fact. They would wake up in the morning and notice that yet another message or picture had been totally or partially removed. They suspected, at first, that their dog was to blame, but this explanation was soon discarded as infeasible.

Because of the "refrigerator incident," coupled with the fact that they heard so many strange noises, the women finally concluded that there was indeed a ghost in the house. This, it seems, was not something they wanted to think, but something they could no longer deny. One night, while staying in the house alone, Ruth was woken up at about three o'clock in the morning "to this insane racket in Carol's room." It sounded, she said, "like someone was just picking her iron bed up and throwing it on the floor."

One stormy, rainy night, while Ruth and Joan were watching TV in the living room, they heard "a prominent loud knock" on the front door. At that time, the front door wasn't connected to its hinges, and therefore wasn't being used, but was simply laid up against the doorway. All of their friends realized this, and everyone entered and exited the house via a different door. The fact that the house was situated on a hill with a long driveway leading up to it meant that, if someone had driven up to the house, Ruth and Joan would have seen the light from their car's headlights. But there were no cars to be seen or heard, least of all any people.

When Joan said "come in," no one answered. They then heard the knocking sound again. "And at that time we both just sort of freaked out," said Ruth. Their hearts beating frantically, they switched on all the lights in the house and ran into the kitchen, where Joan armed herself with an axe and Ruth a knife. From the kitchen, they heard the sound of what they thought was the front door opening. That it actually physically opened would have been impossible, of course. Creepier still, they also heard footsteps in the hallway, "and we weren't going to wait around any longer to find out who it was, or what it was!" said Ruth. The women exited the house via the back door and ran directly to a neighbor's house, where they telephoned some friends who eventually arrived to pick them up. That same night they returned to the house with a couple of male friends, "and we made them go through every room. And there was nothing there. There was nothing strange about the house at all."

Rather than spend that night at the house, Ruth and Joan decided to stay at a friend's place. From that day forward, they were well and truly frightened of being in the house, whereas before the disturbances has only made them anxious. According to Joan, living in the country by themselves was not a big deal for her and the others, as they had been doing so for years, and they considered themselves to be a fairly brave and resilient lot. It's fair to say that anyone in the same set of circumstances would have been afraid, no matter how brave or unimaginative. It would not be unreasonable to suppose, moreover, that the ghost was trying to create an atmosphere of fear in the house, so as to drive the women out.

Not long afterwards, the women invited some friends over for a group water coloring session. One of the guests painted a creature that looked like a "demon." It was, said Carol, "a horrible looking picture." That night, the demon from the paining made an appearance in one of Carol's dreams. In it, Carol remained terrified as she was chased by the demon through a huge, spacious building.

The women soon agreed that action needed to be taken to combat the haunting. The house had become almost uninhabitable, and they did not want to continue living in fear. As is sometimes the case in these matters, someone claiming to be a great occultist or medium decides to lend a helping hand, usually for ego gratification more than anything else. This time was no exception. A fellow student named Jack, a self-proclaimed medium who was "really heavy into the occult," approached the women. He was, said Ruth, "really eager to help. I think he was too eager."

There was little doubt in Carol's mind that Jack was a phony, but this didn't stop the women from accepting his "help." Jack, the young Aleister Crowley wannabe, told Carol that she was a witch, and that she was partly responsible for the haunting. After subjecting the women to an ESP test, he went into a fake trance in which he pretended to communicate with several spirits. The spirits must have been an uncooperative bunch because they did not materialize before him as requested. Before leaving, Jack left an amulet in the house (of the magical kind, presumably) and asked if he could return at a later date to hold a séance. Jack was never invited back, and the women never spoke to him again.

Ruth wasn't the only one in the house to be attacked by the ghost while asleep. The same thing happened to Carol. She along with the others had gone to bed at around one o'clock. A couple of hours later, she was woken up "by this real, hysterical, cackling laughter." She began to puzzle over who was responsible for the noise, thinking, initially, that it may have been Joan and Ruth. As she lay in bed, still half-asleep, her attention was drawn to an odd rustling sound coming from the direction of the stairs.

Carol explained what happened next: "And then I smelled this really foul odor...And then my bed starts rocking sideways, making this insane racket...And then I was touched on the neck and in the shoulder area... And from that point outward I just tingled all over. And again I couldn't move and I couldn't scream. Until I finally thought the word 'No!' And as soon as I thought, 'No!' I thought, 'I can't fight this.' And then it went away."

Once out of bed and fully awake, Carol was unable to find any evidence that a dog had entered the room, or had defecated or urinated in the room – which is what she initially suspected to be the cause of the unpleasant smell. The possibility that a person had come into the room was also out of the question, she says. It should be remembered, by the way, that although Carol's experience would nowadays be classified as an SP episode, she did not have a label to assign to her experience at the time the interview was conducted in 1974, nor was she aware of Hufford's research into the Old Hag phenomenon. In short, she was completely ignorant of the very existence of the phenomenon, as were Ruth and Joan. I cannot stress this enough.

The experience left Carol in a state of shock. She ran downstairs to Joan's bedroom, situated directly below hers. Joan explained to Carol that she had not heard the sound of laughter, although she had heard a "thumping" noise coming from upstairs, which was so loud it had woken her up. Was this, perhaps, the sound of Carol's bed rocking sideways? (Once again, one wonders if Carol's bed had actually moved at all. Perhaps it had been an "illusion" created by the ghost, the sound of which had been artificially generated, as was clearly the case when the front door was heard to open.)

That same night, the ghost made its presence known again; all three women heard footsteps coming from upstairs in Carol's room. The footsteps travelled down the stairs and onto the front porch. Then they heard the screen door slam shut.

Because Ruth and Carol were too scared to sleep alone, they now slept together in the same bed, with the light switched on all night. Joan, however, was not afraid to sleep alone, and, unlike Ruth and Carol, she didn't mind being in the house on her own at night – at least not too much. "And I was just at the point in my head that I wasn't going to be driven out of my house by this ghost," she says. One evening, while suffering from a virus, Joan went to bed quite late, before Ruth and Carol returned home from work. She then "woke up" to a "bad dream" at four o'clock in the morning. But, she says, it "wasn't like waking up."

While in a state of paralysis, she saw a series of images in her mind's eye. The experience, she says, was like watching a TV screen in her mind. "It wasn't," she insists, "like a dream...It was like you were made to watch these things going on before you...Like I was watching a TV documentary or something, of all these horrible killings...So I was trying to reject it. Just eject it out of mind, but I couldn't. And then it started getting heavier... Then I started seeing these axes flashing through the air! And I saw myself, like it was urging me to do something evil. It was like a power..."

As the "power" tried to possess her, Joan felt a pleasant tingling sensation enter her body, eradicating the pain and discomfort caused by the virus she had contracted. "And then I just felt good." She tried to force herself out of bed but still could not move. Eventually, however, she managed to wake herself up. Satisfied that the "power" had left her, she decided to drift back to sleep. But this proved to be a mistake. Within fifteen minutes, "I could feel it again...I felt like it was urging me to do something I didn't want to do." She saw, once again, a "picture show" in her mind. "I was watching myself murder Ruth and Carol!" She saw herself wielding an axe, chopping Ruth and Carol into pieces.

As she struggled once more to resist the "power," the tingling sensation returned. In her interview with Hufford, she described the sensation as having an inward quality, rather than an external one. Having felt the same sensation, Carol was able to add: "It's like your nerve ends are just all being stimulated by some real pleasant vibration or something." The tingling, said Joan, is accompanied by a "heaviness" or "pressure" in one's chest, which spreads throughout one's body "until you just can't move...or like you just don't *think* about moving really...Because it feels *good*." (I, too, have had this experience, and would describe it in much the same way.)

According to Joan, the intensity and persistence of the "power" was such that she had to "fight it off" a total of three times. Knowing that she would not be able to resist it a fourth time, that she did not possess the strength to do so, she jumped out of bed and ran up the stairs to Carol's room where Carol and Ruth were asleep. Without waking them up, she lay down in the spare bed. She stayed awake for the remainder of the night, "just kind of staring, just petrified," while listening to the ghost call out her name. She also heard a strange moaning sound, the sound of someone breathing, and even sensed a presence in the doorway. Asked why she chose to endure the experience, and why she didn't wake up the others, Joan said "it wasn't in my mind to do it...I don't know. I was supposed to go through it or something."

By the time the presence had gone and the disembodied noises had ceased, morning had arrived. "The night was one of horror," said Joan. The ghost, she stressed, had influenced and overpowered her mind, causing her to act in a passive manner. As she explained to Hufford: "I felt like it was trying to control me...That it wanted to overcome my will. That it was intent on either doing something to make me...I don't know...freak out mentally...Or it wanted me to do something evil physically." Joan left the house for good that day, never to sleep there again.

With Joan gone, Carol and Ruth's fear of living in the house increased. One evening after arriving home from work, they were surprised to discover that several lights in the house, including the porch light, had been left on – or rather, had been *turned on*, for they were certain they had switched them off before heading out that day. Before they had the chance to switch the porch light off, or indeed any of the lights, it mysteriously turned off by itself. Spooked, Carol and Ruth left immediately, staying the night at a friend's place. Following this incident, the usual disturbances continued with regularity. One of the ghost's favorite pastimes was to call out their names – and this it did quite frequently. And at night, it would often produce loud banging sounds.

When someone suggested to the women that a Roman Catholic priest might be able to help, the idea appealed to them, even though they were not religious. The priest listened carefully to what they had to say but initially seemed very skeptical. Nevertheless, he visited the house to conduct a blessing ceremony, leaving behind a crucifix, some holy water, and a candle. But soon after he left, the holy water mysteriously disappeared, and Ruth and Carol were unable to find it anywhere in the house. At first the women were convinced that the ceremony had been a success. The ghost, they thought, had finally left the house, and now they could live in peace.

In actual fact, the ghost had not gone anywhere. It was just as determined as ever to drive them out of the house, and now it had only two people to deal with. One night, while lying down to go to sleep, Carol noticed that she couldn't move. She then felt something touch her body. When, at last, she was able to speak, she frantically called for Ruth, who dashed upstairs to check on her. Ruth, along with a friend named Bill, ended up sleeping in Carol's bedroom so as to comfort her. Ruth and Bill slept in the bed together, and Carol slept on the couch.

That night, Bill had a disturbing "dream" during which he was unable to move. He described it to the others as a "recurring dream," adding that the last time he had had it was about fifteen to seventeen years ago. Bill was firmly convinced that the occurrence of the "dream" – or recurrence, rather – was directly linked to his being in the house.

Bill and Ruth woke up around six o'clock the following morning and went downstairs, while Carol remained asleep. A couple of hours later, Bill heard moaning sounds coming from Carol's bedroom. When he dashed upstairs to see if she was okay, he noticed she was still asleep. According to Carol, Bill then shouted, "You are all crazy! You are crazy for living here! Get out!" His words must have had an impact because Carol and Ruth did not stay in the house much longer. The attack on Carol – the one that occurred the night Bill stayed over – was the final straw.

Since leaving the house, Carol and Joan told Hufford, their physical and mental health had improved, and they generally felt much better. While living at the house they had "been at each other's throats" most of the time, and their friendship had deteriorated. But moving had fixed all this, and they felt just as close as ever.

Hufford's interview with Carol and Joan revealed that both women, before they had moved into the house, had experienced at least one SP attack each. (Though, of course, they did not refer to these experiences as "SP attacks," or, for that matter, "Old Hag attacks," for they had no knowledge of either phenomenon.) These experiences, they believed, had been caused by malevolent spirits. They described them, moreover, in much the same way as the ones they had experienced while living in the house. Asked by Montell whether she believed in ghosts, Carol said, "I've experienced them before." She then proceeded to tell him about two "ghostly encounters" she had had many years ago, one of which deserves mention here.

At age eighteen or nineteen, Carol had been invited to stay with some friends, a couple named Frank and Rose, who lived on a 1000 acre farm – "a little community" – consisting of seven houses. She arrived there around nine o'clock at night accompanied by a male friend. Exhausted from the long drive, she decided to have an early night. Frank and Rose's house was large and old with two spare bedrooms upstairs. Carol chose the bedroom she preferred the most. Soon after she lay down in bed, the door handle began to jiggle, and then the door opened. No one entered the room or was standing at the doorway, so Carol thought the wind must have blown it open.

Looking back at the doorway, she saw a "bright shimmering substance," a "very vaporous-looking thing" float over to the foot of the bed. She could hear it breathing heavily, even when she held her breath. "And I couldn't move. I was just s-s-scared stiff. Paralyzed! And whatever it was came around to the side of the bed and walked behind my back. And I'm straining my eyes trying to see it, but I can't move my head…"

Carol felt a strange tingling sensation travel up and down her spine. Meanwhile, images of a knife began to flash through her mind, "and I thought, 'My God, I'm going to be stabbed in the back with a knife.'" She then felt pressure on the bed, felt it sink down as though someone were sitting on it. The pressure was suddenly released as "whatever it was" moved over to the foot of the bed and "hovered there for awhile." As it exited the room, Carol saw the door close behind it. Feeling "exhausted and limp," she knew the attack was over and that the ghost would not return. For a moment she heard the rocking chair in the hallway rocking by itself, "and I knew there was a ghost outside the room," but she no longer felt so afraid.

The following morning, Carol reported the incident to Rose, explaining that there appeared to be a ghost upstairs. Rose confessed that she and Frank were well aware of its presence, but, because they did not wish to cause her unnecessary alarm, had decided not to mention it. Sometimes, they told her, they'd hear the rocking chair rocking on its own. Or the record player upstairs would suddenly start playing music. According to their landlord, two male friends used to live in the house, one of whom had murdered the other, stuffing his body in a closet upstairs. The body was found four years later. The victim, Carol later learned, had been stabbed in the back with a knife – which is what she had suspected all along. She felt, in fact, that the ghost had been trying to communicate with her and had wanted her to know the manner in which it had been killed – hence the image in her mind of the knife and the thought of being stabbed in the back.

That Carol and Joan had each had at least one SP attack in the past, many years before they'd moved into the house, does not in any way invalidate the assumption that staying in the house somehow contributed to their experiencing more SP attacks than normal. Given the fact that so many other people experienced attacks while staying in the house – such as Ruth and Bill – one cannot deny that the house had a paranormal influence of sorts. What's startling about this case, says Hufford, "is the clustering of so many apparent Old Hag attacks in a single location over a months' time and involving several people...By themselves, these attacks suggest an environmental variable capable of greatly increasing the likelihood of Old Hag attacks."

Of course, when I say "the house" had a paranormal influence, I actually mean the spirit occupying the house. Had the spirit been successfully driven out of the house, then it probably would have been a harmless place in which to live. Those of you who believe in Feng shui, or something similar, might argue otherwise, however. And indeed it's quite possible that certain locations attract, for various reasons, specific types of "energy" of either a malevolent or benevolent nature. Houses built on intersecting ley lines, or above underground streams, are frequently found to be haunted, as many an experienced dowser knows. This, however, is not my area of expertise, and I have few words to offer on the subject.

Although this is difficult to confirm based on the limited amount of information given by the women, it would appear that the house was haunted by not just any kind of ghost but by a poltergeist or "noisy spirit." A definition of the word, as given by *The Penguin English Dictionary*, is: "A mischievous ghost said to be responsible for unexplained noises and throwing objects about." The very fact that most dictionaries contain a precise definition of the word "poltergeist" suggests that its existence is well established, and that many people have encountered such entities. In an article on the poltergeist, Colin Wilson mentions that "they are by no means a rarity; at this very moment some case of poltergeist activity is probably going on within a dozen miles of [where you are at the moment]."

The reason I propose that the ghost of Bowling Green was a poltergeist is that it was able to affect the physical environment, for instance by smearing and removing the paint on the refrigerator. That it was able to interact and communicate with the women in the house – though only to a limited extent – also speaks of a poltergeist, as does the fact that it was able to produce loud noises. The main difference between a poltergeist and a common ghost is that the former is able to move and influence objects, while the latter is not. In most cases, the latter appear to be little more than "psychic video recordings" and not spirits. There are, it seems, many different classes of ghosts, and to describe them all is beyond the scope of this book. All the reader needs to know at this point is that some of them are sentient – i.e. spirits – while others are non-sentient "recordings."

The fact that Ruth's body was extremely cold after she'd just had her first SP attack – the first one to occur in the house – is an interesting observation because there is often found to be an absence of heat in haunted houses, and sometimes, in certain locations, "cold spots" will be present, as though the entity responsible for the haunting has sucked all the thermal energy out of the air. The ghost uses this energy to bring about various physical manifestations, as I'll explain in greater depth later on. For a ghost – a poltergeist, that is – to affect the physical environment in some way, it has to be able to draw energy from any source it can, particularly a living source. And what better source of energy could there be than the aura of a human being in their sexual prime. Could Ruth have felt cold because the ghost had sucked her body dry of vital energy?

As regards the incident in which Carol thought she heard Ruth's bed being thrown around, it was never determined whether the bed actually was thrown around, or if, instead, only the sound of it happening was heard. The possibility exists that the ghost artificially generated the sound. There have been plenty of poltergeist cases recorded in which furniture and other objects have been thrown around and levitated, often in full-view of witnesses. A famous case known as the Enfield Poltergeist is rife with examples of such phenomena. A description of this case is presented in a later chapter.

CHAPTER 6

The Poltergeist According To Spiritism

Poltergeists are manifestations of the unconscious mind – not spirits – according to the popular and "respectable" theory shared by most paranormal researchers. The "spirit hypothesis" is deemed unscientific and sensational, and tends to be avoided like a bad smell. And this, I think, is a great shame.

William Roll's *The Poltergeist* (1972) is among the most significant scientific studies of the poltergeist. Roll, a psychologist and parapsychologist of some note, classifies poltergeist activity as a form of "recurrent spontaneous psychokinesis" (RSPK), noting that most cases involve a psychologically disturbed individual – usually a pubescent child – around whom most of the paranormal activity takes place. This person is usually called the focus. According to Roll, because the incidents occur around a living person, there is no reason to assume that non-physical entities are responsible. "It is easier to suppose that the central person is himself the source of the PK energy," he explains.

But in British author Colin Wilson's view, proponents of the unconscious mind theory, such as Roll, fail to explain "why poltergeist effects are so much more powerful than the kind of psychokinesis that has been studied in the laboratory." A very good point, no doubt, and one that seems to undermine Roll's argument. Wilson, a proponent of the spirit hypothesis, remains one of a very few number of serious paranormal researchers to hold this view.

It's interesting to note that Wilson didn't always support the spirit hypothesis. For many years he preferred to believe that the hidden powers of the unconscious mind could explain the existence of poltergeists. In his book *Beyond the Occult* he tells the interesting story of how he came to adopt a radically different view. It happened, he said, in 1980, when he met the British paranormal expert Guy Lyon Playfair at a conference in Derbyshire, England, where the two of them had been invited to lecture on the paranormal. Because Wilson had made plans to visit a poltergeist investigation following the conference, he asked Playfair, rather casually, what he thought poltergeists might be.

The answer he received rather astonished him. Playfair told Wilson that he thought poltergeists were "a kind of football." Wilson describes the rest of this conversation in his own words: "'Football!' I wondered if I'd misheard him: 'A football of energy. When people get into conditions of tension, they exude a kind of energy – the kind of thing that happens to teenagers at puberty. Along come a couple of spirits, and they do what any group of schoolboys would do – they begin to kick it around, smashing windows and generally creating havoc. Then they get tired and leave it. In fact the football often explodes and turns into a puddle of water.'"

Wilson was, at first, rather critical of Playfair's theory, viewing it as crude and superstitious. But when he arrived in Pontefract that afternoon, at the residence of Mr. and Mrs. Prichard, the location of the poltergeist haunting, he was forced to reconsider his opinion. The first manifestations of the haunting occurred in 1966, at which time, Mr. and Mrs. Prichard's son, Phillip, then aged fifteen, was clearly the focus as their daughter Diane was away on holiday when the paranormal phenomena took place. The activity lasted for a total of two days. When the disturbances began again in 1968, Diane, then aged fourteen, was evidently the focus.

When the poltergeist first arrived, small pools of water began to appear on the kitchen floor. Playfair had told Wilson that these "poltergeist pools" are impossible to make by pouring water onto the floor, as splashing would result – and indeed those found in the Prichard household were unusual and entirely "splash-free." Mrs. Prichard described them as "neat little pools – like overturning an ink bottle." As soon as they were mopped up, explained the Prichards, the pools of water reappeared elsewhere. And when water board officials arrived to search for a leak, none was found. Of course, Wilson was astonished when he heard about the pools of water, as it seemed to corroborate Playfair's theory.

Not only did green foam spurt out of the tap when it was turned on, lights in the house began to switch on and off of their accord, and a pot-plant situated at the bottom of the stairs somehow found its way to the top of the stairs. Wilson observes that the poltergeist seemed to have a sense of humor. On one occasion, in true slapstick fashion, a jug of milk floated out of the refrigerator and poured itself over the head of Aunt Maude, who had earlier revealed her skepticism of the poltergeist's existence.

When in 1968 Diane became the focus, few disturbances occurred during the day while she was at school. During the evenings, however, all hell would break loose. There would be loud drumming noises, ornaments would levitate around the room, and furniture would be thrown around, often smashed. On one occasion, the hallstand made of heavy oak floated through the air, landing on Diane and pinning her to the stairs. Although Diane was unharmed – not even bruised, in fact – moving the object proved to be something of an ordeal, as the family was unable to budge it on their own.

Perhaps the most frightening and dramatic incident that occurred was when the poltergeist dragged Diane up the stairs. It appeared to have one hand around her throat and the other hand on her cardigan. As soon as Phillip and Mrs. Prichard grabbed Diane, the poltergeist let go, and they all tumbled down the stairs. According to Mrs. Prichard, shortly after the incident took place, she found the hall carpet soaked with water and marked by large footprints. Later on, the poltergeist – whom the Prichard's named "Mr. Nobody" – began to manifest visually, appearing as a tall figure dressed in a monk's habit with the cowl over its head. One day Phillip and Diane saw it disappear into the kitchen floor. From that point onwards the disturbances ceased altogether.

A friend of Wilson's discovered that the there had once been a gallows on the site of the Prichard's house, and that a Cluniac monk, convicted of rape, had been hanged there during the time of Henry VIII. The Pontefract case, says Wilson, "left me in no possible doubt that the entity known as Mr. Nobody was a spirit – in all probability of some local monk who died a sudden and violent death, perhaps on the gallows, and who might or might not be aware that he was dead."

This entity, insists Wilson, which seemed to have more in common with a ghost than a typical poltergeist, could not have been a product of Diane's unconscious mind, as the behavior it displayed – such as pulling Diane violently up the stairs – was individualistic in nature. If, indeed, a fragment of Diane's psyche really did split-off, why would it take on the form of a monk, of all things? And why would Diane unconsciously want to create something to scare and torment not only her family but also herself? The question as to why her unconscious mind would want to destroy almost every piece of furniture in the house also begs an answer. "With the exception of Guy Playfair," says Wilson, "there is probably not a single respectable parapsychologist in the world who will publicly admit the existence of spirits."

So how did Playfair arrive at the conclusion that poltergeists are spirits, or, as he likes to put it, "footballs of energy"? To answer this question we need to explore his background. Playfair developed a keen interest in parapsychology in the late 1960s while living in Brazil where he worked as a teacher and freelance journalist. Wanting to learn more about psychic phenomena, Playfair became a member of the Brazilian Institute for Psychobiophysical Research (IBPP), a Spiritist organization founded by the pioneering parapsychologist Hernani Guimaraes Andrade, who passed away in 2003.

Playfair investigated his first poltergeist haunting in 1973. The family, a divorcee and her two children, both of them adults, were troubled by strange disturbances in their home, which had been going on for about six years. The poltergeist produced loud bangs and crashes, set their clothes on fire, and threw furniture around. The disturbances had started, Playfair was told, as soon as the son of the family had married a girl named Nora, leading the family to believe that they had become the victims of a black magic trabalho (work or job). As Playfair explains in his book *The Indefinite Boundary* (1976), the practice of black magic is rife in Brazil, as it is home to many African-influenced cults, two of the biggest being Candomblé and Umbanda, which originated among freed African slaves in the 1830s, and which have their roots in voodoo.

In this poltergeist case, there was plenty of evidence to suggest that someone had been working a black magic trabalho against the family. For instance, a "spirit offering," consisting of bottles, candles, and cigars, was found in the family's garden. Also found on the premises were photographs of a girl with stitches through it – a sign of black magic. The family, it turns out, had many enemies, any one of whom could have organized the trabalho. One of the many suspects was a supposed former lover of Nora's, who may have borne a grudge against her and her husband.

The fact that magic is taken very seriously in Brazil and other parts of the world should not be overlooked. Here in the West we regard such matters as superstitious nonsense. But in many other cultures throughout the world the existence of spirits and other "supernatural" beings is accepted as an irrefutable fact.

The late Andrade – who once called black magic "a really serious social problem in Brazil" – is quoted as saying: "Any Brazilian is well aware that this country is full of backyard terreiros (black magic centers) where people use spirit forces for evil purposes... To produce a successful poltergeist all you need is a group of bad spirits prepared to do your work for you, for a suitable reward, and a susceptible victim who is insufficiently developed spiritually to be able to resist." A suitable reward, according to Playfair, might include any of the following: "A good square meal, a drink of the best cachaca rum, a fine cigar, and perhaps even sexual relations with an incarnate being." In Brazil, says Playfair, even the poorest of the poor will quite happily prepare a magnificent banquet as payment to a spirit (or group of spirits) for doing them a favor.

Fortunately, in Brazil, to combat curses and therefore banish troublesome spirits such as poltergeists, all one has to do is procure the services of an experienced medium, or team of mediums. In Nora's case, a candomblé master arrived at the scene, along with his team of assistants. They performed various "exorcism" rites that appeared to be successful. An earlier attempt to exorcize the poltergeist, which was carried out by the IBPP's poltergeist-clearance team of mediums, was only partially successful in that the disturbances ceased for a period of two weeks then began again. The mediums had apparently asked their "spirit guides" to persuade the poltergeist to leave.

Playfair was a member of the IBPP from 1973 to 1975, during which time he was heavily influenced by the Spiritist ideas of Andrade. And this, of course, brings us right back to the subject of Spiritism. Most people know about the religious movement Spiritualism, which flourished in Europe and America from the 1840s to the 1920s, and whose followers believed, and still believe, that the spirits of the dead can be contacted by mediums. But few of us in the English-speaking world are familiar with the philosophical doctrine Spiritism, which was established in France in the mid-nineteenth century. An offshoot of Spiritualism, Spiritism began with the Frenchman Allan Kardec, whose real name was Hippolyte Leon Denizard Rivail.

Born in Lyon, France, in 1804, Rivail was educated at the distinguished Yverdon Institute in Switzerland, a school founded and run by the famous educational reformer J.H. Pestalozzi. Rivail was so influenced by Pestalozzi and his revolutionary teaching methods that he decided to become a teacher also, eventually establishing his own school in Paris, which, unfortunately, he was forced to close after just eight years due to financial reasons. But Rivail's career as an educator didn't end there. He wrote textbooks on French grammar, mathematics, and educational reform, and also taught free courses in the sciences. Possessed of a great intellect, he apparently spoke six languages. By the early 1850s, writes Playfair, Rivail had become "well-established as a progressive, free-thinking writer and educator." Wilson describes him as "a kind of universal educator, willing to dispense knowledge on any and every topic."

Being, in Anna Blackwell's words, "unimaginative almost to coldness" and "a close, logical reasoner," it's little surprise that Rivail's initial reaction to the Spiritualist "table-turning" craze was one of skepticism. Originating in 1848 with the Fox sisters in Hydesville, New York, the exciting phenomenon quickly spread to Europe. Almost everyone, it seems, was conducting séances in their homes, communicating with the spirits of the dead with the use of a table. In 1854, while discussing the subject with a friend, Rivail remarked, "I will believe it when I see it." He attended his first séance about a year later and was greatly impressed by what he witnessed, which not only included table turning but also a demonstration of automatic writing. "I glimpsed," he explains, "beneath the apparent frivolities and entertainment associated with these phenomena something serious, perhaps the revelation of a new law, which I promised myself I would explore."

Rivail was later introduced to a Mr. Baudin, who held weekly séances at his home. Present at these sessions were his two daughters, both of them excellent mediums. The methods they used to communicate with the "spirit realm" were that of table turning and planchette writing. Because the girls were frivolous and not the sharpest crayons in the box, so to speak, and because mediumship works on the principle that "like attracts like," nothing particularly special was obtained from these communications – except, of course, when Rivail was present. He appears to have acted as a "beacon" for wise and knowledgeable spirits.

No longer were the spirit communications of a banal and superficial nature. The spirits began to talk philosophy of "a very grave and serious character," and Rivail used the opportunity to ask them the most penetrating questions he could think of. He came to each session with a list of new questions. Examples include, "What is God?", "Do spirits foresee the future?", and "Is it possible for man to enjoy perfect happiness upon the earth?" Their answer to the first question was simple yet elegant. God, they said, is "the Supreme Intelligence – First Cause of all things." Rivail, by the way, was not a medium himself, and thus he relied on others to act as his "telephone line" with "the other side."

Another group of researchers, no doubt as earnest and sincere as Rivail and his colleagues, also conducted numerous "question and answer sessions" with apparently wise and knowledgeable spirits, in the end collecting more than fifty notebooks full of compelling material, which they ended up handing to Rivail. He added it to the other communications he had obtained himself. Overall, the information seemed entirely logical and possessed an impressive inner-consistency. That it had a profound impact on Rivail, spiritually, intellectually and philosophically, is proven by the following statement, which he made to his wife: "My conversations with the invisible intelligences have completely revolutionized my ideas and convictions. The instructions thus transmitted constitute an entirely new theory of human life, duty, and destiny, that appears to me to be perfectly rational and coherent, admirably lucid and consoling, and intensely interesting."

After two years of scrutinizing the material, Rivail decided that it might be a good idea to collate, edit, and publish it. When he asked his "spirit communicators" what they thought of the notion, they replied in the affirmative, giving him specific instructions as to how he should go about it: "To the book...you will give, as being our work rather than yours, the title of *Le Livre des Espirits* (*The Spirits' Book*); and you will publish it, not under your own name, but under the pseudonym of Allan Kardec." ("Kardec" was an old Breton name in his mother's family.)

Rivail spent a considerable amount of time organizing and verifying the communications. He only wanted to publish the best and most credible material – credible in the sense that the information could be confirmed by a number of different "sources," and that it fitted in with the overall "theme" of the work. If he wasn't satisfied with the answer to a question – perhaps because it conflicted with the rest of the information he had collected – he would submit the question again, sometimes to a different medium than the one he had originally consulted. Rivail's method, although not perfect, was certainly far more credible than that of most people who receive communications from the "spirit realm" and who are often willing to believe almost anything they're told.

The Spirits' Book was finally published in 1857 and caused quite a stir. It was so successful, in fact, that a second addition containing additional material was printed the following year, and the name Allan Kardec became known all over France. That its "author" was a respected intellectual – and not the sort of person one would expect to publish such material – astonished the public. Almost everyone was able to find something of value in the book, even those of a scientific disposition, as it deals with such a wide range of topics in a very intelligent and enlightening manner.

According to Steve Hume in an article that appeared in *The Noah's Ark Review*, the French working classes took to Spiritism the most, "perhaps for the simple reason that the spirits had nothing good to say about the inequity that was, and still is, inherent in human society." He points out, for instance, that the Spiritist teachings utterly condemn selfishness; proof of this can be found in *The Spirits' Book*, which reads, "It is from selfishness that everything evil proceeds. Study all the vices, and you will see that selfishness is at the bottom of them all."

Few can deny that *The Spirits' Book* is an impressive piece of work and that much food for thought can be found within its pages. One might describe it as an attempt to answer many of the "big questions." As well as the nature of God, some of the topics it covers include the purpose of life, the origin of spirits, human ethics, the afterlife, and spiritual evolution. Some of the information is ahead of its time. On the topic of "universal space," for instance, we are told than an absolute void does not exist in any part of space, but that "what appears like a void to you is occupied by matter in a state in which it escapes the action of your senses and of your instruments." It's exciting to think that "quantum field theory" (QFT), which postulates the existence of a "quantum vacuum," did not originate until the 1920s – more than half-a-century after the publication of *The Spirits' Book*. According to QFT, in an article available on Wikipedia, "the vacuum state is not truly empty but instead contains fleeting electromagnetic waves and particles that pop in and out of existence."

In chapter VIII of *The Spirits' Book*, the question is asked: "Do spirits influence our thoughts and our actions, and to this the reply is given: "Their influence upon them is greater than you suppose, for it is very often they who direct both." In chapter IX the book explains that spirits are incessantly around us, "and when you fancy yourselves to be hidden from every eye, you often have a crowd of spirits around you, and watching you." Fortunately for us, however, the book also explains that spirits can only see us if they choose to do so, and if they direct their attention towards us. Therefore, if we don't attract their attention and their interest, they'll happily leave us alone, for a spirit "pays no heed to those which do not interest him."

In addition to *The Spirits' Book* are four other fundamental works, also written – or, in Rivail's words, "compiled and set in order" – under the name of Allan Kardec. They include *The Mediums' Book*, *The Gospel According to Spiritism*, *Heaven and Hell*, and *The Genesis According to Spiritism*. All five books – known collectively as *The Spiritist Codification* – were published before Rivail's death in 1869. Playfair describes them as "the clearest and most comprehensive survey of the invisible world yet written."

The major difference between Spiritualist doctrine and Spiritist doctrine is that the latter advocates reincarnation, while the former does not. This had the effect of dividing the two movements. The spiritualist teachings, of course, came into being through automatic writing and table turning – not trance mediumship. Automatic writing was the type of mediumship most favored by Rivail, who considered it among the safest, describing it as a method "by which the spirits best reveal their nature, and the degree of their perfection or inferiority." The Spiritualists, on the other hand, were, and still are, fond of practicing trance mediumship, while most of their mediums – or, rather, the spirits speaking through them – mentioned nothing at all about reincarnation. For this reason, explains Wilson in his book *Poltergeist!*, "Rivail was inclined to be critical about trance mediums, while the trance mediums and their followers denounced Rivail as a dogmatic old man."

Following Rivail's death in 1869, Spiritism essentially died out in France and the rest of Europe, and, before long, his name was just about forgotten. Although the movement never took root in Europe, perhaps because it was too conservative a culture both religiously and scientifically, the Brazilians embraced it with open arms. And, in 1873, the Society of Spiritist Studies was formed in Rio de Janeiro. From then on, Spiritism continued to flourish, to the point where today, according to the last IBGE census data, more than four million people declare themselves "Kardecist Spiritists." Furthermore, although the majority of Brazil's population is Catholic, it is estimated that around 20 million people *believe* in Spiritism and benefit from it. "In short," writes Hume, "Spiritism in Brazil is a vibrant religious movement that gives hope, comfort and inspiration to millions who would otherwise have no relief from...poverty..."

Spiritism teaches us that man is made up of three entities – the spirit, the body, and the perispirit. The perispirit is basically another name for the astral body and is described as a "semi-material envelope...drawn from the universal fluid of each globe." When we die, the physical body is left behind, but the spirit remains united to its perispirit. It acts as a bond between the physical body (material) and the spirit (immaterial). "On account of his ethereal nature," explains *The Mediums' Book*, "a spirit cannot act upon gross matter without an intermediary, that is to say, without the link which unites spirit to matter; this link, which is what you call the perispirit, gives you the key to all the materialized spirit-phenomena." We are told that the density of the perispirit varies from spirit to spirit, and that the more highly evolved the spirit, the more ethereal its perispirit will be. Apparently, spirits who have "attained perfection" no longer need their perispirits.

In chapter V of *The Mediums' Book,* an in-depth – and entirely plausible – explanation of the poltergeist is given. Poltergeists are classified as "imperfect spirits" trapped in materiality. Some are downright evil and dangerous. Others are boisterous, noisy, and mischievous, though not necessarily malevolent. It is in the latter category that poltergeists best belong, for very few of them actually harm their victims.

The person around whom the disturbances take place – the focus, in other words – is described as being an "unconscious medium," in the sense that their presence is necessary for the poltergeist to manifest itself. (The SP sufferer is also a kind of "focus" for discarnate entities.) Although a spirit is able to act to some extent upon matter, it requires extra energy (vital fluid) to do so and must draw this energy from a living person – i.e. a medium. The poltergeist combines its energy with that of the medium's, thus enabling it to manipulate the physical environment – which is something it could not do on its own.

Considering that poltergeists are said to make use of the focus's energy without their realization or consent, it would not be unreasonable to classify them as a type of "vampire." If the focus manages to bring their mediumistic powers under control, states *The Mediums' Book*, then it's likely the disturbances will cease.

CHAPTER 7

The Enfield Poltergeist

Of all the poltergeist cases that have been recorded over the centuries, one in particular continues to interest me – and indeed many other paranormal enthusiasts – not only because it makes for a frightening, dramatic, and entertaining story, but because it provides great insight into how these disturbances are created and how they operate. By studying the Enfield case, one is able to gain a basic understanding of the "physics" behind poltergeist disturbances and consequently the "physics" of SP attacks.

The first manifestations of the haunting began on August 30, 1977, at the home of single mother Peggy Hodgson and her four children: Margaret, thirteen; Janet, eleven; Pete, ten; and Jimmy, seven. The house, located in the suburb of Enfield, North London, was a place of much activity, as the children were often boisterous; young children normally are. It was also a place of considerable despondence, as Mrs. Hodgson had recently separated from her husband. The atmosphere in the house was far from happy.

Pete and Janet shared the same bedroom. That evening, soon after they had gone to bed, something shook their beds in a way that defied explanation. When they told their mother what had happened, she thought they were playing games. She told them to go back to sleep.

The next evening, the children heard a strange shuffling noise, as did Mrs. Hodgson. They also heard four loud knocks. Then things got truly bizarre. They all watched in amazement as a heavy chest of draws slid out from the wall on its own. As soon as Mrs. Hodgson pushed it back into position, it slid back again. When she tried pushing it again, the object wouldn't budge. Something was preventing it from moving. Scared out of their wits, everyone rushed downstairs. Mrs. Hodgson told her neighbor Vic Nottingham about the incident, and he agreed to go inside and take a look for himself. He searched the house from top to bottom, attempting to find out what had caused the strange phenomena. But he was just as baffled as everyone else.

Typically in poltergeist disturbances, the victims are bothered by loud and persistent knocking sounds. This case was no exception. As soon as the lights were switched off, the knocking started. The sound emanated from different areas of the house and would often shift around from wall to wall.

Sometimes it would come from the ceiling.

That same night, the police were called in to investigate. Naturally, they found it difficult to take the case seriously and were unable to offer any assistance. Just as they were preparing to leave, however, the poltergeist decided to "show itself." A chair levitated off the floor and began moving across the room. According to WPC Carolyn Heaps, "it came off the floor nearly half an inch. I saw it slide off to the right about four feet before it came to rest. I checked to see if it could have slid along the floor by itself. I even placed a marble on the floor to see whether it would roll in the same direction as the chair. It didn't. I checked for wires under the cushions and chairs and I could not see any. I couldn't find any explanation at all."

The following evening, the disturbances began again. The poltergeist started hurling small objects, like marbles and Lego bricks, around the room. One of the marbles that had been thrown was found to be hot to the touch. A friend of Mrs. Hodgson's called up the *Daily Mirror*, which sent a reporter and photographer to investigate the paranormal activity. Once again, objects began flying around the room at great speed. The photographer began snapping pictures frantically, eager to capture the paranormal activity on film. During the commotion, a Lego brick flew across the room and hit him on the brow; the bruising lasted a few days. Referring to this incident in his book *Poltergeist!*, Wilson calls it "one of the few examples of a poltergeist actually hurting someone."

When the photographs were later developed, they were found not to exhibit any poltergeist activity whatsoever. All they showed were terrified and astonished witnesses. The poltergeist, it seems, had tried to make sure its actions were not caught on film. Everything it did must have taken place just outside the range of the camera.

Wanting to help the distraught family, the *Daily Mirror* decided to contact the Society for Psychical Research (SPR). The first SPR member to arrive at the scene was Maurice Grosse, whose daughter, Janet, had recently died in a motorcycle accident. He had joined the SPR shortly after her death; the reason, according to some, is that he desperately wanted to find proof of life after death. The other SPR member who decided to offer a helping hand was Playfair, who would later pen a successful book on the Enfield Poltergeist entitled *This House is Haunted* (1980). He and Grosse would end up being involved in the case for about two years.

During the course of their investigation, Playfair and Grosse witnessed and documented all sorts of strange phenomena. Ornaments floated in mid-air; objects mysteriously disappeared, only to reappear later in odd locations; pools of water suddenly showed up on the kitchen floor. And of course there were the ghostly noises, like those knocking sounds, which sometimes emanated from inside walls as well as from the floor. "I was quite intrigued by the way they seemed to come from all parts of the floor at once, as if several different knockers were at work," explains Playfair. "Some were loud, some soft, *and some sequences would fade in and out like a weak radio signal*" (my emphasis). Footsteps were also heard. The intelligent, lively, and athletic Janet was quickly identified as the main focus, an assumption that proved to be correct.

On one occasion, Playfair saw a marble land on the floor from far away. When it struck the smooth linoleum surface, however, it didn't roll in the slightest, as it should have according to the laws of physics. Playfair tried to duplicate this inexplicable effect but found it impossible. On another occasion, to see how the poltergeist would react, Playfair tied Janet's chair and bed together using wire. When he inspected it several minutes later, he found the wire had been snapped and the chair toppled over. When he tried the "experiment" again, the same thing occurred. It was then that the poltergeist began to get rowdy. An armchair tipped over; then the bed shot across the room. A book, appropriately titled *Fun and Games for Children*, flew off the bookshelf, landing upright on the floor. Their attention was then drawn to one of the pillows on the bed, upon which they saw the indentation of a small head, as though an invisible person was resting there.

The poltergeist continued to knock on a frequent basis. One time it did so for two and a half hours, leading Playfair to conclude that it wanted to communicate. To facilitate the process, a medium named Annie Shaw was invited to the house, along with her husband George. Annie went into a trance and was supposedly "taken over" by an entity. She screamed "Go way," began to cackle, and even spat at George. She then uttered the words, "Gozer, Gozer, help me. Elvie come here." George confronted the "entity" that was speaking through his wife and told it to leave the family in peace.

Once out of the trance, Annie told the others that Janet was indeed the focus of the poltergeist activity, as previously established. She said that several entities were behind the haunting. One of them, she added, was an old woman. As for "Gozer," George described him as a "nasty piece of work, a sort of black magic chap," and he said that "Elvie" was "an elemental." Annie said that Janet's aura was leaking energy and that her mother's was too. When this happens, she explained, poltergeists are able to steal one's energy, which they use for their manifestations.

The cause of the "leakages," said Annie, could be attributed to the negative atmosphere in the house, which was brought about by the separation of Mrs. Hodgson from her husband and the pent-up bitterness she felt towards him. Before leaving, Annie and George performed an aura healing exercise on Janet and Mrs. Hodgson. This seemed to help because the poltergeist went quiet for a period of several weeks. When it returned, however, it behaved more violently than before. While working at the house one morning, Playfair became aware of a "tremendous vibrating noise."

"I really thought someone was drilling a great big hole in the wall of the house," he explained. "I tore into the bedroom and there was quite a commotion. The whole fireplace had been ripped out. It was one of those old Victorian cast-iron fires that must have weighed at least 60 lb. It was so heavy even I couldn't pick it up. The children couldn't have possibly ripped it out of the wall. It just wasn't possible. We caught the incident on audio tape, including the fireplace being ripped out of the wall."

Eventually, Playfair tried communicating with the entity himself, using a code: one rap for "yes" and two raps for "no." Paying no attention to the code, the poltergeist rapped thirty times in a row in a very angry fashion. "Once again," says Playfair, "*they sometimes faded and came back just like a radio program from a distant station*" (my emphasis). When he asked, "Don't you realize that you are dead?" the poltergeist became upset. Loud crashing sounds could be heard coming from one of the upstairs bedrooms. The poltergeist, it turns out, had completely trashed the room, scattering objects all over the floor.

That the poltergeist had a personality of sorts is evidenced by the fact that it liked some people and disliked others. It had taken a definite dislike to Playfair but didn't seem to mind Grosse. When Grosse tried communicating with the poltergeist, it cooperated to some extent. When he asked it if it had died in the house, it knocked once, indicating "yes." The entity claimed to have lived in the house for more than thirty years. After a while, the poltergeist began to answer Grosse's questions in a nonsensical fashion. "Are you having a game with me?" he asked it. Before he had time to blink, Grosse was struck in the forehead by a box containing cushions. Instead of flying across the room, the box appeared to vanish from its original position, then rematerialize a split second before hitting Grosse's head.

Wanting to communicate with the poltergeist further, they asked it to write out a message on a piece of paper. They left a pencil nearby. When they returned a few minutes later, somebody or something had written the following words on the piece of paper: "I will stay in this house. Do not read this to anyone else or I will retaliate." Mrs. Hodgson forgot about the "warning" and showed the message to her ex-husband, who had come to drop off his maintenance money. She then apologized aloud to the poltergeist. Soon afterwards, another message written on a piece of paper appeared on the table. "A misunderstanding," it read. "Don't do it again. I know who that was."

Janet, meanwhile, was not having an easy time. The poltergeist had her under its spell. When attempting to get to sleep, the poltergeist would often throw her out of bed, or yank the blankets violently off her body. One night the poltergeist tried to stifle her, placing a "hand" over her mouth and nose. When Janet finally managed to get to sleep, she would often twitch, moan, and cry, as though under possession. On one occasion, after being thrown out of bed, she went into convulsions and started screaming hysterically. Restraining her proved to be something of a struggle, as she exhibited a frightening amount of strength. The following night, Janet went into convulsions again, and, while in a trance state, began wandering around the house, saying out aloud, "Where's Gober? He'll kill you."

In December 1977, the poltergeist began making whistling and barking sounds. Then it began to speak. The voice said its name was "Joe Watson." In response to the question, "Do you know you are dead?" Grosse was angrily told to "Shut up." When Playfair tried reasoning with the poltergeist, explaining that he and the others were only trying to help, the voice growled "Fuck off." Its voice could best be described as being like that of a drunken old man, though it also had a slight electronic quality to it. It refused to speak when the investigators were in the room. Furthermore, it seemed to be incapable of talking politely and would frequently use obscene language.

The voice finally said its name was "Bill." It said it kept shaking Janet's bed because "I was sleeping here." Bill said he enjoyed annoying everyone in the house. "I am not a heaven man," he explained. "I am Bill Haylock and I come from Durant's Park and I am seventy two years old and I have come here to see my family but they are not here now." Bill said he "had a hemorrhage and then I fell asleep and I died in a chair in the corner downstairs." Subsequent research revealed that a man named Bill – last name Wilkins, not Haylock – had died in the house. He died, moreover, in exactly the same way the voice described – of a brain hemorrhage while sitting in a living room chair downstairs. Bill Haylock, it turns out, was a former local resident – a neighbor, in fact.

The voice continued to make rude remarks. On one occasion, when Margaret tried asking a question, it became furious, calling her a "fucking old bitch." It then said: "I want some jazz music. Now go and get me some, else I'll go barmy." Another time, Grosse's son, Richard, came to the house. "You're a Jewish rabbi," the voice said rudely. Indeed the Grosse's were Jewish, but Richard was not a rabbi. "Why, are you afraid of them?" Richard asked the voice. The voice replied: "They're always praying their heads off." Interestingly, observed Playfair, "whenever the subject of God, religion or prayer came up, the voice would react strongly and become abusive or, as in my brief experience, refuse to communicate altogether."

Although the voice came from Janet – and was obviously connected to her in some way – she did not appear to be entirely responsible for its production – at least not consciously so. This was confirmed by an experiment Grosse conducted, in which he made Janet hold water inside her mouth. To make absolutely sure she couldn't talk, he also sealed her lips together with masking tape. With all these measures in place, the voice could still be heard. "The voice is so obviously that of an old man that the notion of Janet producing it by ventriloquism is absurd," wrote Colin Wilson in *Poltergeist!* For a short period of time, the voice issued from Margaret as well, sounding very similar to the one that came from Janet. Asked what she felt when the voice "spoke through" her, Margaret replied: "Just the vibrations in my neck, as though it was right behind me."

Physics Professor John B. Hasted, known for his research on paranormal metal bending, concluded that the voice was being produced by the "false vocal cords," or ventricular folds, and not the standard vocal cords. The former play no part in normal speech. A very small number of people, however, are able to speak using their false vocal cords but only for very short periods of time; to do so requires great effort, and because there isn't sufficient liquid to lubricate the false vocal cords, they become inflamed very quickly, giving you a sore throat. How the voice was produced both by Janet and Margaret remains a genuine mystery.

Shortly after the poltergeist started speaking, Janet was seen to levitate above her bed. Two independent witnesses observed the event: a lollipop lady and a baker, who happened to be glancing up at Janet's window when it occurred. According to Janet, now aged 41, "The lady saw me spinning around and banging against the window. I thought I might actually break the window and go through it. A lot of children fantasize about flying, but it wasn't like that. When you're levitated with force and you don't know where you're going to land it's very frightening. I still don't know how it happened."

Even though the haunting had been going on for a while, the poltergeist had not yet given up. Perhaps because it wished to keep its audience guessing, it began to produce all sorts of new phenomena. It started fires, created horrible smells, and smeared ordure on the walls. It even wrote obscene messages on the bathroom mirror, such as "shit" and "I am Fred."

That the children were responsible for some of the paranormal phenomena is already well established. The two main culprits were Janet and Margaret. "They weren't very good at playing tricks," recalls Guy. "We always caught them out. What do you expect children to do? I would have been more worried if they hadn't played around from time to time. It means they were behaving like normal kids." Out of the many hundreds of paranormal events that took place in the house, Janet says she and Margaret were responsible for very few – around two percent, according to her estimate.

According to two Brazilian Spiritist mediums who visited the house, Janet had been involved in witchcraft during a previous lifetime and was now being punished for her actions. One of the mediums wrote: "I see this child, Janet, in the Middle Ages – a cruel and wanton woman who caused suffering to families of yeomen – some of these seem to have come back now to get even with her and her family."

Another medium, named Gerry Sherick, was of much the same opinion, claiming that both girls had once dabbled in witchcraft. While in a trance state, Sherick began to channel a sinister old woman, whom he believed to be connected to the haunting. Using a voice that was not his own, Sherick said: "I come here when I like… I'm not bleedin' dead, and I'm not going to go away." Before leaving, Sherick performed psychic healing on the family members so as to repair the leaks in their auras. Once again, the disturbances ceased for a while, then returned. Another factor that rendered the poltergeist less energetic was Janet's stay in the Maudsley Hospital, a psychiatric institution in South London. She was taken there for observation and testing in mid-1978, and her health improved as a result.

A Dutch medium named Dono Gmelig-Meyling claims to have been responsible for finally bringing the haunting to an end. After visiting the house, he went on an "astral trip," and met the spirit of a 24-year-old girl. The girl was thought to be Grosse's daughter, Janet, who would have been 24 if still alive. Dono sensed she was connected to the haunting in some way. But he did not think she was responsible for any of the poltergeist activity.

That the case involved two "Janets" is certainly an interesting coincidence, if nothing else. Playfair speculates that the spirit of Grosse's daughter had intervened in some way, so that her father would become involved in the case. As for Dono, it's quite possible that his "astral intervention" is what brought the haunting to an end. But this is impossible to prove. During a recent interview, Janet remarked: "I know from my own experience that it [the poltergeist] was real…It lived off me, off my energy. Call me mad or a prankster if you like. Those events did happen. The poltergeist was with me – and I feel in a sense that he always will be."

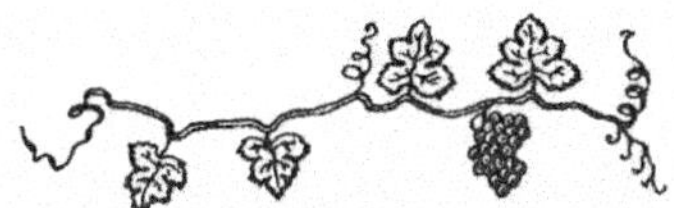

Let us now analyze the case and search for any clues that may help us better understand the SP phenomenon. First of all, it's clear that the spirits responsible for bothering and interfering with humans are of a imperfect nature, and that there are many different classes of imperfect spirits, just as there are many different classes, or types, of people, some nice, some mean, etc. *The Spirits' Book* classifies spirits into three different classes: Imperfect Spirits, Good spirits, and Pure Spirits. It is only the first class that concerns us here, which is broken down into five principal subcategories: Impure Spirits, Frivolous Spirits, Noisy and Boisterous Spirits, Neutral Spirits, and Spirits Who Pretend to Know More Science than they Possess.

The general characteristics of imperfect spirits are as follows: "Predominant influence of matter over spirit. Propension to evil. Ignorance, pride, selfishness, and all the evil passions which result from these." Under the topic of Noisy and Boisterous Spirits, it is written: "They often manifest their presence by the production of phenomena perceptible by the senses, such as raps, the movement and abnormal displacing of solid bodies, the agitation of the air, etc. They appear to be, more than any other class of spirits, attached to matter…" Clearly, poltergeists are imperfect spirits and best belong in the noisy and boisterous category. Most – if not all – of the spirits responsible for SP attacks are of an imperfect nature also.

In the Enfield case, it's obvious that more than one spirit was involved. Following the separation of her parents, an event that caused the family a great deal of stress and unhappiness, a group of spirits – perhaps as many as ten – attached themselves to Janet. A number of mediums who visited the house said that Janet's and her mother's auras were leaking energy –

which the poltergeist was using for its manifestations. After they'd had their auras "cleaned," the disturbances ceased for a short period. The poltergeist then was indeed an "energy vampire," as are most of the spirits responsible for SP attacks. It would not be unreasonable to conclude, moreover, that those most open to possession by unwholesome spirits are emotionally disturbed or sexually frustrated in some way. Janet was probably suffering from anxiety and depression. That she had just reached puberty should also be taken into consideration.

During the course of the haunting, Janet behaved as though she were under possession, especially when asleep, whereby she would sometimes twitch and moan. She was also given to trance states and convulsions, as is common among poltergeist agents. This is interesting when you consider that some SP attacks are an *attempt at possession* by discarnate entities, and that these attacks occur while you are asleep and your "psychic guard is down." You could say that Janet was possessed by the poltergeist at all times – that is, for the entire duration of the haunting – but that the poltergeist was able to possess her to an even greater extent while she was asleep and vulnerable.

Imperfect spirits, being "strongly attached to the things of this world, whose gross satisfactions they regret" and having a "propension to evil," are constantly wandering the "earth plane" in search of people whom they can influence and exploit. Their victims would be those who are open to "psychic attack," people who, because they are depressed, anxious, or sexually frustrated, are leaking vital energy from their auras. Attracted to the "scent" of this energy, a spirit or group of spirits would then home in on its source, creating trouble for their incarnate victim.

In the case of a poltergeist disturbance, it would mean that the spirit (or spirits) have successfully managed to possess their victim, and are harnessing their victim's energy to create various types of manifestations – e.g. the levitation of objects, the production of loud noises, etc. On the other hand, in the case of an SP attack, it would mean that the spirit's (or spirits') attempt at possession was unsuccessful, or that they only wanted to steal their victim's energy, nothing more.

Before we continue, there is one small matter I need to clarify, which involves my use of the word "possession." Some might think it inaccurate to use this word in regards to the position of the agent, by saying that they are "possessed by the poltergeist." And this I can understand, for it could be said that the agent is not fully "taken over" by the poltergeist. However, given the fact that the agent is an unconscious medium who's been taken advantage of by a spirit, and that this entity is working through them without their full consent or knowledge, it would not be unfair to say that that a spirit has possessed them. Those keen to split hairs may prefer to use the word "obsession." According to Spiritist doctrine, there is no such thing as spirit possession in the true sense of the term; rather it should more accurately be called "spirit assimilation." Instead of possessing a person – which is apparently impossible – a spirit assimilates himself to someone "who has the same defects and the same qualities as himself, in order that they may act conjointly." This is an interesting point to consider.

In the Ghost of Bowling Green case, it would appear that the spirit occupying the house wanted to possess at least one of the three women – which is why they all experienced SP attacks – and that, had it been successful, a typical poltergeist disturbance would have erupted with one of the women being the focus. The entity was unable to become a full-blown poltergeist (assuming it was a kind of poltergeist) because it didn't manage to harness enough energy. It failed, in other words, to acquire a focus, perhaps because neither of the women was a powerful enough medium or maybe because their wills were too strong for it to overpower. The agent, remember, is an unconscious medium, and without an agent there can be no poltergeist; for a poltergeist to enter our reality, so to speak, it needs someone through whom it can work and through whom it can bring itself into being.

The women found these encounters so terrifying and traumatic that they decided to leave the house, and no wonder, because their experiences matched those of rape victims. They literally felt that the ghost was trying to take over their minds and bodies. So powerful was the entity's grip on Joan's mind that she felt as though "it was trying to control me." She then realized "that I had to get away. That I wasn't strong enough to overpower it." And who knows, had it successfully overcome her will, maybe she would have ended up harming Ruth and Carol.

To recapitulate, there are, I think, many different types of spirit possession; being the agent of a poltergeist disturbance is but one type. SP attacks, on the other hand, could best be classified as an attempt at possession, although this does not apply to all such attacks, for they vary greatly in nature. It's quite likely that certain spirits attack people in their sleep, not because they wish to possess them as such, but because they wish to feast on their vital energy. The evidence seems to suggest, moreover, that all imperfect spirits are energy vampires to some extent.

The incorporeal beings who interfere with humans and create suffering are generally troubled and lacking in spiritual knowledge, and are sometimes referred to as "earth bound spirits." Ghosts, of course, would belong in this category, the poltergeist in particular. An occultist would say that these entities are still attached to earthly pleasures, that their desires have shackled them to the ground, that they have, in a sense, become trapped.

In Joe Fisher's chilling investigation into channeling and spirit guides, *The Siren Call of Hungry Ghosts* – which we'll explore in the next chapter – he makes a comparison between these "earth bound spirits" and the Tibetan Buddhist idea of "hungry ghosts" or *pretas*. The belief in hungry ghosts is common to many religions, primarily Buddhism. These poor wretched souls with their enormous distended bellies, long thin necks, and narrow limbs are said to exist in a state of constant hunger and suffering, their appearance being a metaphor for their mental condition. They have enormous yet totally insatiable appetites, hence their large bellies and thin necks. Those who in life are overcome by jealously and greed are believed to run the risk of being reborn as pretas. Although normally invisible, they can under the right conditions be perceived by humans. According to some traditions, pretas are a lot like demons, in that they are able to shape-shift, use magic, and also have a craving for human blood.

CHAPTER 8

Mediumship, Channeling, And The Joe Fisher Story

When spirits begin to speak with man, he must beware lest he believe them in anything; for they say almost anything; things are fabricated by them, and they lie; for if they were permitted to relate what heaven is, and how things are in the heavens, they would tell so many lies, and indeed with solemn affirmation, that man would be astonished...They are extremely fond of fabricating: and whenever any subject of discourse is proposed, they think that they know it, and give their opinions one after another, one in one way, and another in another, altogether as if they knew; and if man then listens and believes, they press on, and deceive, and seduce in diverse ways. – Emanuel Swedenborg, *Spiritual Diary*, 1622

When it comes to encounters with "hungry ghosts," no story is more disturbing and tragic than that of Canadian journalist and best-selling author Joe Fisher. Fisher committed suicide at age 53 on May 9, 2001, throwing himself off a limestone cliff at Elora Gorge, Canada. His body was discovered by a group of teens. One newspaper suggested he may have been murdered. Shortly before his death, Fisher's final book, *The Siren Call of Hungry Ghosts*, an investigation into channeling and spirit guides – described by its publisher as "his gripping journey into a realm of darkness and deception" – was republished by Paraview Press. What gives this story a strange twist is that, in one of his last communications with editor Patrick Huyghe, Fisher stated that the spirits he had allegedly angered as a result of writing the book were still causing him trouble.

Fisher's works include the metaphysical classics *Life Between Life*, *Predictions* and *The Case for Reincarnation*, the last of which includes a preface by the 14th Dalai Lama. In an article on the topic of "spirit possession," Colin Wilson, who acknowledges Fisher as a friend, mentions that he "had been cheerful and normal, and no one, including myself, could believe that he had killed himself." He mentions, moreover, that Fisher believed in life after death and subscribed to the theory of reincarnation. "What baffled me was that he must have been convinced that suicide would only leave him with another set of problems."

Wilson has a point, because in *The Case for Reincarnation*, Fisher had written: "Those who learn that they have killed themselves in past lives are quickly brought to the realization that suicide, far from being an answer to life's problems, is [instead] the violent breaking of the lifeline. If the [suicide] could only realize the resulting intensification of difficulty which must enter the life to come, [suicide] would never be [attempted]."

That Fisher's death was caused by a group of malevolent discarnate entities – who perhaps influenced his mind – might sound far-fetched and sensational. It is, however, a possibility that cannot be ignored as anyone who's read *Hungry Ghosts* would probably agree. Unable to accept that an optimistic, spiritually-minded man like Fisher would want to take his own life, Wilson writes: "I find myself speculating whether his suicide had anything to do with a weird experience he had in the 1980s."

That "weird experience" began in 1984, when Fisher met an Australian-Canadian medium named Aviva Nuemann, who suffered from chronic leukemia. Aviva had contacted Fisher, suggesting he attend a channeling session at her house because, she said, she did not feel entirely comfortable being a "mouthpiece" for discarnate entities and was hoping that he, an expert on metaphysics, might be able to shed some light on the matter. When they first met, Aviva, a laboratory technologist, stressed the point that she had "never believed in the so-called psychic world. I think astrology is absolute crap, and I've got no time for anything that's supposed to be paranormal…" She then told him the remarkable story of how she became a channeler for "the guides."

It all started, she said, when she agreed to allow her friend, Roger Belancourt, to try and heal her under hypnosis. His aim was to administer positive medical suggestions to her subconscious mind, such as "Your bone-marrow will start immediately to manufacture the extra red blood cells needed by your body." These hypnotic sessions took an experimental turn when Roger began probing Aviva's mind for past-life memories. In an emotionless voice in the third-person, Aviva described having been a peasant woman named Svetlana who lived through the Russian revolution, as well as a Punjabi infant who died of malnutrition before his first birthday. Other "past life memories" were described as well.

Probing deeper still, Roger managed to contact another part of Aviva's mind, even more knowledgeable than her subconscious. It referred to itself as the "alter-consciousness." Roger discovered that every organ of Aviva's body, and every aspect of her personality, appeared to possess its own alter-consciousness, each with its own voice. He used the "voices" to monitor Aviva's health. By communicating with the blood's alter-consciousness, for instance, Roger was able to tell whether Aviva's red blood cell count had increased or decreased. This higher aspect of Aviva's mind – what one might term her "superconsciousness" – proved to be very knowledgeable about spiritual matters. The aim of reincarnation is "forward development," it said, which is "understanding of oneself."

When brought back to full consciousness, Aviva had no memory of what had transpired while in trance. It was as though she had been deeply asleep. "Coming back isn't much fun," she told Fisher. "It's as if I'm being dragged very swiftly up a mineshaft…it's like hearing an alarm go off when I'm dead to the world." Seeing as her alter-consciousness seemed to know just about everything, Roger decided to ask it if "spirit guides" actually existed for he had long suspected that he was watched over by a deceased Tibetan Lama named Jai-Lin. Roger found to his delight that he could communicate with Jai-Lin via Aviva's alter-consciousness, which in Fisher's words "acted as intermediary, relaying messages from the next world." His "guide" told Roger that he "must always think positive thoughts," and that "you have much to learn in self-discipline."

Annoyed by the fact that Roger was unable to control his negative emotions, Jai-Lin told Roger that he must move on to meet fresh challenges elsewhere. Jai-Lin was eventually replaced by another "guide," an affectionate entity named Hanni, who claimed to have been Roger's mother in a previous life in the Netherlands. Every incarnate individual was administered a spirit guide, Roger was told. But this did not necessarily mean that one had the same guide throughout the whole course of one's life – or, for that matter, several life times. Sometimes a guide would leave their "charge" – the incarnate person whom they were required to "watch over" – and another guide would fill their place.

Having mastered the ability to manipulate Aviva's vocal cords – a process that was said to take some time – Hanni was able to speak through the entranced Aviva. Fisher describes Hanni's voice as "soft and tenderly" and totally dissimilar to Aviva's. While channeling her own guide – a Yorkshire farmer named Russel who claimed to have last lived on Earth during the 19th century – the voice that issued from Aviva's mouth was also unlike her own, so much so that it left Fisher stunned. "Gone was the high-pitched jocularity with the pronounced Australian lilt. Her enunciation was now unequivocally masculine; the English accent was unmistakable."

Speaking to Russel, Fisher was not only surprised by Aviva's change in voice but by her change in personality, too. "This was an entirely different Aviva," he says, "strangely assertive and uncompromising." Fisher felt as though he were talking to a separate being and not a fragment of Aviva's unconscious mind. Russel told Fisher that humanity was divided into two groups: souls and entities. Souls were said to be "created from desire," while entities were "born of knowledge." Neither group was superior, said Russel. Although he found the concept difficult to accept, Fisher was glad to be hailed as an entity – clearly the more appealing of the two groups. Entities were classified as individuals, while souls were said to have more of a group mentality.

Fisher's guide turned out to be a young Greek woman named Filipa Gavrilos. Three centuries earlier, said Russel, she and Fisher had been lovers in a little Greek village called Theros. Apparently they had been together over many lifetimes. The news blew Fisher away as he had always been strongly drawn to Greece, and, as a child, the name Phillipa had appealed to him. Russell described Filipa as an "excitable young lady." Eventually, he said, she would be able to speak through Aviva. In the meantime, Fisher tried to develop mind-to-mind contact with Filipa, something she had encouraged him to do. Each day, Fisher would close his eyes and will Filipa to communicate with him, a regimen he followed religiously for the next three years.

It didn't take long before a small group of New Age enthusiasts had gathered around Aviva, all of them eager to communicate with their guides. Regular sessions were held every week. No guide was available for those who were classified as souls, because the souls of guides, it was said, occupied a separate and inaccessible plane to that of entities. In late 1984, Filipa spoke through Aviva for the very first time. Fisher describes her voice as "subdued, pensive and poignantly tender."

Initially, admits Fisher, he was rather unimpressed with Filipa and had "serious doubts about her intelligence…Her initial responses were almost juvenile, prompting me to remark to Roger and Aviva that I had attracted a 'disco queen' for a guide." As the sessions continued, however, Filipa quickly became "an advisor, a best friend. And my ideal lover." He adds: "Filipa and I seemed to think alike, feel alike and see the world from a near-identical perspective."

What complicated the situation is that Fisher had a girlfriend, named Rachel, who also attended the meetings, though very infrequently. Her guide, William, spoke with a thick Scottish accent and claimed to have last lived in Edinburgh during the 17th century. They had strong karmic ties, he said, having shared more than twenty lifetimes together. Fond of William though she was, Rachel couldn't help but feel slightly repulsed by him and the other guides. "For all their signs and wonders, the guides gave her the creeps," writes Fisher. While in their presence, she sometimes felt "a certain intangible negativity in the air..." She eventually dropped out of the group, and, in time, she and Fisher drifted apart. He had, after all, found a more suitable partner in Filipa – non-physical though she was – who "knew and understood me more precisely than anyone..."

The guides said they could read the minds of their charges, which seemed to be true. They knew certain things about their charges that only their charges knew. They could, for instance, describe what their charge had been doing or thinking on a particular day and at a particular time – information that could only have been gained psychically.

Every so often, said the guides, it was necessary for them to intervene directly in the lives of their charges. One time Aviva had driven through a snowstorm to collect her six-year-old son from school, despite the fact that Russell had warned her not to, claiming it was too dangerous. She arrived safely at the school. But for some strange reason her car wouldn't start on the way home. Several drivers gave her a boost, and still the engine wouldn't respond. "But," she told Fisher, "as soon as the snowstorm abated, the engine started perfectly, as if nothing had happened." Questioned about the incident later on, Russell claimed responsibility for the temporary engine failure. Had he not intervened, he said, Aviva would have had a potentially fatal accident on the way home.

Fisher's daily attempts to communicate with Filipa on a mind-to-mind basis began to yield some interesting results. Whenever contact had been successfully established, "a loud buzzing would reverberate in my ears, a sound that could be likened to an internal droning of cicadas." (One is reminded of Mary's "critter" experiences.) During these meditative sessions, images would sometimes appear in his mind. One time he saw the image of woman walking towards him. She was wearing sandals and a long white wrap, her face partially hidden by a garment. He knew the woman was Filipa. "Within seconds, my body was racked with the most profound and unrestrained emotion. I wept out of joy and sadness and loss and anguish, yet to this day I don't really know why."

Mind-to-mind contact could best be achieved when Fisher was in a particularly relaxed mood, with very few thoughts running through his head. Sometimes he'd imagine himself hugging Filipa, and this she appreciated greatly. Fisher could tell that she longed for a physical body. "I wish that I could stand there and wipe your face and hold your hand," she told him on one occasion. Filipa and the other guides disliked nothing more than to be referred to as "spirits" and to be reminded of the fact that they no longer occupied physical bodies. To call one of the guides a spirit was to annoy them, even make them angry. "We're not spirits!" Russell once shouted. "We're people just like you. It's just that we don't have bodies anymore." Fisher found it a little dubious that the guides were so attached to the "physical plane," even though they stressed that they were no more "spiritually evolved" than their charges.

Occasionally, said Fisher, conversations with Filipa "would erupt in my head." Once, while running up a steep hill, Fisher heard "a voice or implanted thought-form." So as to make the climb much easier, the "voice" told him to imagine that his feet were not touching the ground. The technique had a positive effect. When next at Aviva's house, Fisher asked Filipa if she had spoken to him while he was out running. She answered yes, and was able to relate exactly what she had told him. "Somehow," explains Fisher, "Filipa had to be either living inside me or hovering perpetually close by, picking up via some otherworldly antenna my organism's every twitch and shudder."

In a sense, alludes Fisher, he was able to interact physically with Filipa and even have sexual intercourse with her. During a private conversation with Fisher, Wilson asked him if he "meant they [he and Filipa] became lovers in the physical sense, and he said yes, he did. I felt it would tactless to ask exactly how they went about it."

The guides appeared to have access to an almost unlimited amount of information. They even claimed to know "the nature of God." However, they said, the amount of time required to explain it would take some three hundred sessions; for this reason, the project was never attempted. Fisher admits to being impressed by the teachings and advice offered by the guides. They were taught, among other things, about the history of Atlantis and Lemuria; about the workings of the mind; about reincarnation, karma, and spiritual development. And so on and so forth. "So rich and so abundant were the insights and observations that there were times when I felt overwhelmed by the veritable geyser of information," he says. Communicating with the guides was an addictive and thrilling experience.

But as time went on, Fisher grew slightly suspicious of the guides. When, during one session, Filipa said she was aware of every thought he ever had about her, "the remark left me weak with ardent appreciation. *Every time I thought of her, she knew*. How attentive, I asked myself, can you get?" The guides gave long lectures about the importance of peace and love, but in many ways their teachings rang empty and possessed little substance. Also worrying was that they intervened, both physically and emotionally, in the lives of their charges, while at the same time stressing the importance of free will. Such a massive contradiction was impossible to explain.

In his book *The Paranormal*, British psychologist Stan Gooch – whose research is detailed in the next chapter – describes the teachings of "spirit guides" as "a kind of intellectual candy-floss...when you chew on these utterances, there is nothing there. The mouth is empty." The late D. Scott Rogo, a prolific writer and researcher of parapsychological phenomena, was of much the same opinion as Gooch. "I find that most channeled discourses possess the spiritual and philosophical sophistication of a Dick-and-Jane book," he explains in *The Infinite Boundary*. He once tried reading the Seth books, he says, "but I eventually found raking up the leaves from my mulberry tree more interesting and spiritually enhancing."

At times the guides made statements that were just plain ridiculous, one of them being that Jesus Christ was no more "spiritually evolved" than any member of the group. Russell even stated that Jesus has "been back to the earth-bound many, many times." According to him, the only reason that Jesus managed to achieve what he did is because he spoke the truth, and because he lived during desperate times when people needed someone to follow. As for Guatama Buddha, he hadn't, to the best of Russell's knowledge, reincarnated since.

"The more I loved Filipa," writes Fisher, "the more I hungered for tangible proof of her existence." For this reason, coupled with the fact that he wished to write a book about discarnate beings and life in the "next dimension," Fisher set about trying to prove the identities of the guides. He wanted to know if they had lived the lives they said they had. Fisher knew enough about spirits to realize that they were rarely who they claimed to be. He had, in fact, been warned about this by Russell, who, during one of their first conversations, stated clearly that mischievous spirits sometimes like to pose as wise and knowledgeable spirit guides.

The guides were more than happy with Fisher's desire to prove their identities and were eager to offer him specific details about their lives on earth. First of all, decided Fisher, he would try to follow up on the information given by ex-RAF bomber pilot William Alfred Scott, the guide of a man named Tony. Scott said he had been born in Bristol in 1917, had started his RAF career in 99 Squadron at Mildenhall, Suffolk, and, ironically, had not been killed in the air but in a German bombing raid on Coventry in 1944. Scott knew everything about the squadron, its operations, and his fellow officers. But Fisher discovered, after a visit to the Public Record Office at Kew, that there had been no Flying Officer William Scott in the Squadron.

One surviving member of the Squadron, Norman Didwell, who listened to a recording of Scott's voice, confirmed that the man had never existed but said that his voice sounded "very, very familiar." In addition, the alleged place of Scott's death – a street called Sandrich – was found not to exist. Numerous other details were found to be bogus too. Before leaving England, the country of his birth, Fisher paid a visit to his mother, a devout Christian. "You're talking to demons," she told him. "And I don't like the sound of it one bit."

When back in Canada and in a bitter mood Fisher confronted Scott as to why he had lied, the once calm and polite entity became peevish and irritable. "I do not wish for my privacy to be violated," he said. "I have given you all the information you need and, as such, it will stand." Worming his way out of the situation, Scott claimed that he was unable to stick around for very much longer because he had made plans to reincarnate soon. A suitable "bodily vehicle" had been located in Southern England, he said. After saying farewell, Scott allegedly departed for the "physical plane." Much later on, Russell provided details of Scott's "new incarnation" – his name, DOB, place of birth, and the names of his parents. Surprisingly, the information checked out, and Fisher managed to obtain a birth certificate for the infant. Fisher contacted the parents, who, although intrigued by the matter, were unwilling to get involved. He respected their decision.

Attempts to verify Russell's last incarnation on Earth also met with failure and disillusionment. The same was true of a guide named William Harry Maddox, who claimed to have fought and died during World War I. The war records proved that Maddox had never existed. Fisher's research, by the way, was absolutely impeccable, as can be expected from a former investigative journalist with many years experience. He searched every nook and cranny for evidence of the guides' lives. Why it is that some of the information they provided was true, while the crucial facts from their stories were missing, did not make the least bit of sense. If the guides had wanted to be believed, thought Fisher, wouldn't they have claimed to be people who had actually existed? Were they, perhaps, drawing on the knowledge and memories of other people – either living or dead – to create their identities?

As for his beloved Filipa, she too was found to be a liar and deceiver – or, in Fisher's words, "a master of deception." During his travels through Greece, Fisher was unable to find the ruins of Theros, let alone any evidence that the village had actually existed. And not only that, the city of Alexandroupolis, which Filipa had mentioned visiting during the 18th century, had not even existed at that point in history. In fact, Fisher discovered, the city had been named after a 20th century monarch! "I felt like crying for the group of believers in Toronto, for the guides themselves, whoever they were, for the elaborate deception in which I had become entangled, and for all the all-enveloping, myopic struggle of incarnate life," he writes.

During the remainder of his stay in Greece, while lying in bed late at night and brooding on Filipa's betrayal, "her buzzing returned to plague me. Once so comforting and reassuring, the noise in my ears took on a shrill and sinister aspect, leaving me sleepless." At that point, says Fisher, he began to grow afraid of Russell, Filipa, and the other guides. "If they knew us all so intimately – as they had demonstrated on countless occasions – who could say what power they wielded over our lives?"

In *Hungry Ghosts*, Fisher describes having confronted Russell several times about his lying and manipulative ways, as well of those of "his cronies," and how, because of their remarkable intelligence and their vast understanding of human psychology, such efforts were totally futile. During one "interrogation," the group's "transcriber," whom Fisher describes as a "slavish apologist," leapt to Russell's defense again and again. She was unable to accept the possibility that the guides were even capable of lying. The information needed to prove their identities must be out there somewhere, she insisted.

After the guides had been unmasked, only one or two members left the group. Overall, their faith in the guides had hardly been shaken. Fisher describes Russell – clearly the leader of the guides – as "devious, manipulative and potentially dangerous" and "as slippery as the proverbial eel and a master psychologist to boot." Fisher was unable to talk to Filipa because, said Russell, "You've quite completely shut her out." They never spoke again. In an article on the Joe Fisher story, the philosopher and paranormal investigator Jonathan Zap suggests that the guides may have actually been "a single shape-shifting entity who, like the devil, 'hath power to assume a pleasing shape' and was capable of performing a whole cast of characters of both genders."

An-ex member of the group, Sandford Ellison, told Fisher how the guides had almost ruined his life. During private sessions with the guides, particularly with Russell, Ellison was told that if he didn't leave his wife – a soul, not an entity – he would die. They even said that she was trying to kill him "by projecting powerful negative energies" his way. While working with the guides who were teaching him to channel "healing energies," Ellison suffered from "fierce emotional fluctuations and bouts of muddled thinking." When no longer in their presence, he felt much better. During his final conversation with Russell, when he explained that he wanted nothing further to do with the guides, Ellison was told "*that I would commit suicide in a fit of depression*" (my emphasis). Before splitting with the guides, Fisher, like Ellison, had felt poorly. "I was more jittery than usual," he says, "more susceptible to insomnia and nervous tension…I could not shrug off a cloying sense of contamination which could neither be pinpointed nor explained."

Having spent years listening to, and talking intimately with, the entities channeled through Aviva, and having spoken with a number of other channeled entities, Fisher was forced to accept, somewhat ruefully, that these ostensibly wise and benevolent beings – "who have wormed their way into that juicy apple of spiritual regeneration known as The New Age" – were nothing more than "lower astral entities" or "hungry ghosts." Ellison also concluded that the "guides" were "lower astral entities," adding that they "play on human frailty and feed on our energy and our emotions."

While investigating the channeling phenomenon (which attracted far more attention during the 1980s than it does now), Fisher befriended a woman named Claire Leforgia, a former nursing assistant who apparently channeled her own spiritual teacher – or guide – an English surgeon from the 19th century named Dr. Samuel Pinkerton. Called "wise" and "adorable" by those in the Toronto New Age community, Pinkerton sometimes "spoke so sweetly that it was hard to tell whether his politeness was genuinely considerate or gloatingly sarcastic," says Fisher. Fisher eventually concluded that the charming Dr. Pinkerton was yet another hungry ghost posing as a benevolent guru. Attempts to verify his identity were met with failure; Dr. Pinkerton was not who he claimed to be.

When Fisher mentioned to his friend Alexander Blair-Ewart, editor of the Canadian New Age periodical *Dimensions*, that Dr. Pinkerton enjoyed smoking cigars and drinking alcohol through Laforgia – whom he sometimes referred to as his "instrument" – he was told: "Spirits like Pinkerton get a rush by swooping into a body and satisfying themselves with the sensations of physical life – sensations such as drinking alcohol, for example. This is contrary to the teachings of all the great spiritual masters. This is forbidden. *This is possession, not true spirituality*" (my emphasis).

In the 2001 edition of *Hungry Ghosts*, which contains an epilogue not available in the original edition, Fisher relates a chilling story that might help explain the cause of his suicide. Early in 1988, he says, while living in a small house near Lake Ontario and planning to write *Hungry Ghosts*, he developed a strange abscess on his navel. Each doctor he visited "was equally mystified by the inflammation." Taking antibiotics did nothing to cure the infection, which got progressively worse and tremendously painful. The third doctor he saw, a wilderness specialist – "a man who had seen everything" – told Fisher "I've never seen anything like it." After treating the infection, he assured Fisher that it would heal in time.

Weeks later, alone, and during the middle of winter, Fisher realized that the infection was only getting worse, and that he needed to take emergency action. He was in so much agony that he had to swallow a strong painkiller every half-an-hour. "*Perhaps, I mused, I was under some kind of psychic attack* [my emphasis]. Were the various entities, who had ultimately failed to win me over, trying to ensure I would not reveal who they are and what they do?"

Sometime after midnight Fisher climbed into his car and drove twenty minutes to the nearest hospital, hunched over the steering wheel in pain. He was escorted to the emergency ward and given an injection of Dermatol. An ultrasound revealed that he had omphalitis, a condition in which the umbilical cord becomes infected. Rare in adults, omphalitis usually affects newborns and is most likely to occur to those with abraded, ulcerated, or unclean navels. None of these stipulations applied to Fisher, thus it was a complete mystery as to how the abscess had formed. Due to the severity of his condition, Fisher was operated upon within hours of having checked in. After all, he was told, it can sometimes happen that the accumulated pus explodes internally, leading to peritonitis and even death. Fortunately, the operation was successful.

In what sounds like something out of the paranormal thriller *The Mothman Prophecies*, Fisher received, about an hour after the operation, a mysterious telephone call from Laforgia, who inquired as to his condition. When he asked Laforgia how she had known he was in hospital – for no one had been notified of his admission – she said that Dr. Pinkerton had informed her. That Dr. Pinkerton had attacked him psychically, giving him omphalitis, is a possibility that Fisher was unable to ignore. He writes: "The site of the abscess was symbolic indeed; the navel, the very core of my being." Following his recovery and while working on *Hungry Ghosts*, Fisher was in a state of almost constant paranoia – and perhaps understandably so: "Even if my onetime friends ultimately found a way to take my life, I told myself, the book must be finished."

In his aforementioned article on "spirit possession," Wilson asks the question: "Was his suicide an attempt to rejoin Filipa?" To support this theory, Wilson explains how Fisher's involvement with Filipa had "spoiled him for a normal sex life," as revealed in the following quote, taken from *Hungry Ghosts*: "My terrestrial love life was doomed. No woman of flesh and blood could hope to emulate Filipa's love and concern. No incarnate female could ever begin to understand me in the fashion to which I had become accustomed. In a sense, I was lost to the world, living in a limbo land..."

Wilson offers another compelling theory: "I talked about the mystery of Joe's suicide to Suzanna McInerny, who is the president of the College of Psychic Studies in South Kensington. Suzanna confirmed that long-term involvement with 'hungry ghosts' can cause difficult inner problems. A kind of dirt sticks to the medium's 'aura' (or vital energies), which has to be cleaned off by another medium, like a window cleaner polishing off grime. This dirt can cause depression and a sense of unreality. And sometimes, Suzanna said, a 'hungry ghost' can even hang around inside somebody, quite unsuspected, and can only be evicted by a medium who understands such matters. She agreed with me that this could well be the explanation of Joe's suicide."

Fisher was of the opinion "that no highly-evolved, spiritual being would ever speak through a medium." He quotes the late Tibetan Buddhist lama Namgyal Rinpoche, founder of the Dharma Centre of Canada, who makes the same point: "As a general spiritual law, no enlightened being would speak through an ordinary human. The discarnate spirits who are making themselves known through channeling are united in their desperate need for love. Their audience is a generation that is also hungry for love."

Perhaps Namgyal Rinpoche is right – maybe channeled entities do what they do because they crave the love and attention they receive from their followers. And, although troubled and neurotic, perhaps they're no more harmful than people. Then again, maybe something sinister is afoot. As Jon Klimo suggests in his classic book *Channeling*, the motive behind the channeling phenomenon – for it cannot be denied that most channeled entities are united in a common agenda – may not necessarily be positive but could, in fact, "be offering early warnings of an impending break into a mass psychotic episode, a latter day dark ages with little redeeming value."

In light of Fisher's unfortunate story, it would be easy to form the opinion that all channeled entities are troublesome – possibly even malevolent – lower astral entities, and that, as is written in 2 Corinthians 14, "Satan himself masquerades as an angel of light." For a fundamentalist Christian – which I'm not – such a facile view would be deeply satisfying. But nothing in life is that black and white.

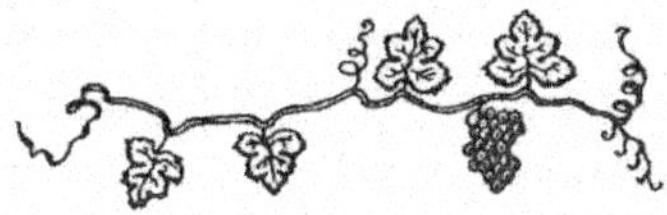

What exactly is channeling, and how does it differ from mediumship? And why do some people criticize the phenomenon, likening it to a form of "spirit possession"? There are, of course, many different forms of channeling, some of them quite safe and not too intrusive – such as various types of automatic writing, for instance. However, the type of channeling investigated and criticized by Fisher is what is commonly called "full trance channeling," whereby the channel, or medium, surrenders their body completely to the non-physical entity who wishes to communicate through them. In most cases, the channeler enters a trance so deep that they remain unconscious during the proceedings. Aviva Neumann was a full trance channeler.

Some researchers make a distinction between the terms "mediumship" and "channeling," explaining that the former involves communication with discarnate humans, while the latter involves communication with all kinds of exotic intelligences, many of them claiming to reside in a separate reality to our own and of a much higher "vibratory level." Another difference is that mediums contact spirits, while channelers are contacted by them. In his article "Channeling: Extrasensory Deception?," the late Suhotra Swami explains this further: "Mediums are experienced clairvoyants who 'fish' for discarnate entities," whereas channelers are "initially psychic greenhorns who, unwittingly or even unwillingly, are taken over by the entities." Please note that the terms "channeler" and "medium" can often be used interchangeably. All channelers are mediums, but not all mediums are channelers.

Channeled entities are not just anyone; they're more "spiritually evolved" than Great Uncle Joe on "the other side" – or at least they profess to be. They include entities like Seth, who spoke through the late Jane Roberts and described himself as an "energy personality essence no longer focused in physical reality." Seth first made his presence known in the early 1960s, when Roberts and her husband began experimenting with an Ouija board – a device known to attract only the lowest class of discarnate entities. Were it not for the publication of Seth's voluminous, intellectual "teachings," channeling would never have gained the popularity that it did – and still enjoys, to some extent.

Before receiving him in light trance then full trance, Roberts could hear Seth's voice in her head. Like so many other mediums, Roberts died at a young age, at 55, in fact, after a long battle with what appeared to be an autoimmune disease. If Seth was indeed a highly evolved being, one can't help but wonder why he felt the need to invade the body of a human being through whom he enjoyed various physical pleasures, such as drinking the odd glass of wine or beer. He even admitted to enjoying the material realm through Roberts's senses.

Prior to coming in contact with Seth, Roberts had a mystical experience of sorts – an experience that opened her up to the channeling phenomenon. It was, she recalls, "as if someone had slipped me an LSD cube on the sly…A fantastic avalanche of radical, new ideas burst into my head with tremendous force, as if my skull were some sort of receiving station, turned up to unbearable volume." The experience Roberts described sounds a little unpleasant, but nowhere near as unpleasant as Australian channeler Shirley Bray's description of how she was first contacted by a group of entities calling themselves "the Nine": "I felt as if thin wires, like acupuncture needles, were being inserted into the base of my skull. It was uncomfortable so I stirred, moving my head from side to side. A voice firmly but gently said, 'Be still, it will not be long.'"

By far the most popular and controversial channeler at work today is the American J.Z. Knight, whose "gift" has earned her many millions of dollars. In 1977, says Knight, while in the company of her husband, she placed a paper pyramid on her head, and "we both started laughing until we cried." The next thing she knew, a "very large entity" was standing before her. "He looked at me with a beautiful smile and said, 'I am Ramtha, the Enlightened One. I have come to help you over the ditch.'"

At Ramtha's School of Enlightenment (RSE), which has attracted some 5,000 students (known as "masters") worldwide and is based in the town of Yelm, Washington, one can learn, according to their mission statement, "the tools and knowledge to tap into the powers of the mind and explore our human potential." One can master remote viewing in just four days, promises RSE, and thus be able to "see the past, present and future of anything at any distance at any time." A weeklong RSE retreat costs about US $1,000. It's estimated, moreover, that Knight's company, JZK Inc., earns a whopping US $10 million per year, perhaps even more.

The less than humble Ramtha describes himself as a 35,000-year-old Lemurian Warrior, who, all those years ago, conquered three-quarters of the world, realized the error of his ways, and quickly gained enlightenment. Ramtha makes no qualms about calling himself a god. We, too, are gods, he says – or, more accurately, "sleeping gods" who have forgotten their true potential. Once we begin to love ourselves, and once we come to realize that we create our own reality, we can achieve anything, says Ramtha. Like many a channeled entity of questionable integrity, Ramtha likes to make dire predictions concerning natural disasters and has even directed RSE students and staff to build underground bunkers stockpiled with emergency supplies. He predicted, in 2000, that 56 square miles of South Sound, Washington, would eventually flood. Ramtha has also predicted earthquakes as well as infections from tainted water supplies.

According to various ex-members of RSE, such as outspoken Yelm-resident David McCarthy who belonged to the organization from 1989 to 1996, Knight is nothing but a cult-leader and a "spiritual predator." The organization, he says, has a small inner circle, to whom its most esoteric Ramtha teachings and pronouncements are revealed – one of them being that the ancient figure Jehovah will return to earth in a spaceship, accompanied by an entourage of flesh-eating "lizard people." Says McCarthy: "A lot of people deny that these things happened. They say these are sacred teachings and that you (outsiders) wouldn't understand."

As was the case with Seth, Ramtha is attached to earthly pleasures and enjoys the occasional glass of alcohol, so much so that he even leads "wine ceremonies." "Many people now speculate that whatever energy came through J.Z. Knight has either shifted, departed, or been replaced by a less benign entity," writes journalist Craig Lee in an article that appeared in the *Los Angeles Weekly* in November 1986.

Were Rivail alive today, it's fair to say that he would probably be highly suspicious of most, if not all, of the entities who speak through channelers, for as we are warned in *The Mediums' Book*: "Repel all spirits who counsel exclusiveness, division, isolation. Such spirits are always vain and shallow; they impose on the weak and credulous by exaggerated praises, in order to fascinate and to domineer over them. As a general rule, distrust all communications of a mystic or fantastic character, as well as those which prescribe ceremonies or eccentric actions."

The Tibetan Buddhists, believe it or not, have mediums of their own. The Tibetan word for medium is *kuten*, which means "the physical basis," and it is through such people that oracles are consulted. Although the practice is rare these days, there used to exist hundreds of oracles in Tibet, probably more. Today there are very few oracles in existence – or, perhaps more accurately, there are very few trained mediums through whom these beings are able to communicate. China's takeover and assimilation of Tibet probably had something to do with this. And, considering that many of these deities were used to assist governmental decision-making and provide intelligence on matters of state, I wouldn't be surprised if the Chinese communist government outlawed the consultation of oracles many years ago.

However, the Tibetan government (that is, the Tibetan government in exile) still consults its oracles from time to time, the principal one being the Nechung Oracle, the main protector divinity of the Tibetan Government and the Dalai Lama. Anyone who's seen the Martin Scorsese film *Kundun*, about the early life of the fourteen Dalai Lama, would remember a rather disturbing scene in which the oracle is summoned and various political questions are put to it, some of them relating to the Dalai Lama's safety. In his autobiography, *Freedom in Exile*, the Dalai Lama confesses that he has dealings with Nechung "several times a year," and that "some Tibetans... have misgivings about my continued use of this ancient method of intelligence gathering." The Dalai Lama describes Nechung as a "wrathful" deity, a "protector and defender." They are, he says, "very close, friends almost." Even so, their relationship is such that "I never bow down to him. It is for Nechung to bow to the Dalai Lama."

In *Freedom in Exile*, the Dalai Lama writes: "Nechung has always shown respect for me...he invariably responds enthusiastically whenever asked anything about me. At the same time, his replies to questions about government policy can be crushing. Sometimes he just responds with a burst of sarcastic laughter. I well remember a particular incident that occurred when I was about fourteen. Nechung was asked a question about China. Rather than answer it directly, the Kuten turned towards the East and began bending forward violently. It was frightening to watch, knowing that this movement combined with the weight of the massive helmet he wore on his head would be enough to snap his neck. He did it at least fifteen times, leaving no one in any doubt about where the danger lay."

When he begins to channel Nechung, the transformation that comes over the medium is a very dramatic thing to watch. The medium's face changes completely, says the Dalai Lama, "becoming rather wild before puffing up to give him an altogether strange appearance, with bulging eyes and swollen cheeks. His breathing begins to shorten and he starts to hiss violently." At the beginning of the ritual, a heavy helmet, weighting approximately thirty pounds (13.6 kg), is tied to the medium's head. In former times, this helmet weighed over eighty pounds (> 36 kg). As to why the helmet was reduced in weight, the Dalai Lama does not say, leading one to speculate that maybe there were more than a few cases of fractured necks.

While channeling Nechung, the medium behaves as though his body were occupied by the devil himself. The process is violent and crass. There can be little doubt that Nechung has no respect for the medium, let alone the medium's body. Trance mediumship, as a general rule, is most exhausting for the medium and in some cases may even be detrimental to their health. This is certainly true when it comes to Tibetan Buddhist mediumship – more so, in fact, than the type of mediumship witnessed in the West, for it is said that kutens live very short lives. According to the Dalai Lama, this can be explained by the fact that "the volcanic energy of the deity can barely be contained within the earthly frailty of the kuten." Assuming this is true, the process could be likened to what happens when the fictional character Dr. Robert Bruce Banner becomes angry and suddenly transforms into the Hulk, his clothes tearing at the seams.

Perhaps the Nechung oracle is nothing more than another deceptive lower astral entity. This is an intriguing thought, and one that very few Tibetan Buddhists would be willing to entertain. That the Dalai Lama, said to be an emanation of Chenrezig, the Buddha of compassion, has been fooled by a "demon" is enough to make one laugh with incredulity. It is, however, a very real possibility, as Fisher's story clearly illustrates.

Thanks to what we know so far about the SP phenomenon, and the ways in which spirits are able to influence the minds of humans, a couple of details of Fisher's story stand out as being of great significance. Firstly, that Fisher achieved partial mind-to-mind contact with Filipa and was able to communicate with her telepathically (though obviously to a limited extent). And secondly, that he was able to have sexual intercourse with her – which, I'm sure, would have occurred on an astral level and which would have been similar in nature to the "succubi" experiences of SP sufferers and others.

Fisher was clearly a victim of spirit possession and to a fairly advanced extent. Being a gentleman, he refused to say much about his sexual encounters with Filipa, which is a shame, I think, because this may have been – probably was, in fact – one of the most important aspects of his relationship with her. Ridiculous though it sounds, they most likely enjoyed a good "astral sex life" and remained closely bonded as a result. Fished stated, remember, that his involvement with Filipa had ruined him for a normal sex life, as pointed out by Wilson.

Perhaps the last word should go to Zap, who warns: "We need to consider the subtle ways that discarnates may influence our thoughts, emotions, sexuality and behavior. Joe Fisher's apparent suicide adds an ominous implication that these entities are not to be underestimated..."

CHAPTER 9

Stan Gooch And The Hypnagogic State

Besides waking life and sleeping life there is a third state, even more important for intercourse with the spiritual world...I mean the state connected with the act of waking and the act of going to sleep, which lasts only for a few brief seconds... At the moment of going to sleep the spiritual world approaches us with power, but we immediately fall asleep, losing consciousness of what has passed through the soul. – Rudolf Steiner, (from the lecture "The Dead Are with You")

Published in 1984, at a time when little was known about the SP phenomenon, is a book by the British psychologist and paranormal researcher Stan Gooch, entitled *The Origins of Psychic Phenomena* (originally titled *Creatures from Inner Space*). The first part of the book deals with SP attacks, or what Gooch refers to as succubi and incubi encounters. Gooch draws a connection between these experiences and poltergeist disturbances, but, being a proponent of the unconscious mind theory, he prefers to believe that spirits, demons, and other entities are nothing but a product of one's own mind, yet are able to take on an objective existence.

The unconscious mind, says Gooch, is far more dynamic and powerful than we assume. It is, in a sense, an entity of its own, possessing its own logic and autonomy, and, when repressed, is capable of expressing itself in very odd and alien ways – poltergeist disturbances being a perfect example. In a balanced individual, he says, the two minds exist in harmony. But when an imbalance occurs, when the unconscious mind is not given its due, there is an externalization of latent energies. It is then that we are haunted by creatures and forces from the mysterious universe of our other mind. Although many of Gooch's views are at odds with those expressed in his book, I feel it necessary to mention some of his findings and experiences.

Born in 1932 in London, England, to a working-class family of Polish descent, Gooch had a difficult childhood. Out of the three children in the family, however, he was the lucky one, as his brother and sister both suffered from a rare and debilitating genetic disease from which they eventually died. His father, a life-long private in the British Army, was physically handicapped, having been seriously injured during the war. Apparently his parents were rather neglectful, and the family lived in squalor. They were eventually moved to a public housing estate. An extremely bright student who read almost every book he could get his hands on, Gooch won a scholarship to a grammar school.

After completing a degree in Modern Languages at King's College, London, he spent a year working in the scrap metal business. The firm he trained with offered him a seat on the board of directors, but he declined the position, deciding instead to work as a schoolteacher. Not satisfied in this profession either, he returned to college and completed a degree in Psychology. He was appointed Senior Research Psychologist at the National Children's Bureau, had numerous papers and articles published in distinguished psychology journals and magazines, and even co-authored an authoritative textbook on child psychology. Being the non-conformist that he was – and still is – and keen to embark on a career as an independent writer and researcher, Gooch had no other choice but to make some huge sacrifices. He not only turned down the position of Director of the National Children's Bureau but also the position of Professor of Psychology at Brunel University, London.

Published in 1972, Gooch's first book (the first one he wrote on his own), *Total Man*, was apparently written in a period of several months and was very well-received, though not as commercially successful as it could have been. It looked as though Gooch was destined to become the next Carl Jung. That *Total Man* was written so quickly can perhaps be explained by the fact that, according to Gooch, it was penned in a state of trance – as were all of his other works. Gooch – as we're about to find out – was a very proficient medium, able to produce automatic writing. However, unlike those who believe that this ability can be attributed to the work of spirits, Gooch asserts, of course, that the unconscious mind is responsible, that automatic writing allows one to tap in directly to the unconscious "storehouse of knowledge."

What followed next was a series of other equally remarkable and original – though slightly more controversial – works, some of which explore topics of a paranormal nature and are extremely underrated and ahead of their time. Some of these titles include *Personality and Evolution* (1973), *The Neanderthal Question* (1977), *The Paranormal* (1978), *Guardians of the Ancient Wisdom* (1979), *The Double Helix of the Mind* (1980), *The Secret Life of Humans* (1981), and *Cities of Dreams* (1989). Never one to have much luck in life and fed up with the fact that he was branded as a kook for his open-mindedness, Gooch retired from writing and went into self-exile in

Wales, where he still lives today – apparently in a rented caravan. Fortunately, however, it would appear that Gooch's luck is finally starting to turn around. Many of his early works are now being republished, and, just recently, he wrote another book, *The Neanderthal Legacy* (2008).

Gooch's involvement with the paranormal began at age 26, when he was working as a schoolteacher in Coventry, England. Because he was new to the area and knew very few people, he decided to enroll in three sets of evening classes, one of which was gymnastics. One evening at gymnastics class, while he was in the changing room, a member of the advanced class named Peter struck up a conversation with him. "He eventually told me that his 'spirit guide' had instructed him to do so." Peter, a spiritualist and medium, invited Gooch to a séance at his parent's house.

The séance comprised eight-to-ten people seated on hardback chairs facing the medium. Soon after it commenced, Gooch had an experience that was to change the direction of his life. At first he felt light-headed. "And then," he explains in his book *The Paranormal*, "it seemed to me that a great wind was rushing through the room. In my ears was the deafening sound of roaring waters. Together these elements seized me and carried me irresistibly forward. As I felt myself swept away I became unconscious."

When he regained consciousness, Gooch was told that several entities had spoken through him while he was in a trance state. One of the entities identified himself as a cousin of Gooch's who had been killed in World War II. Told by the presiding medium that he was a "strong natural medium" and that he ought to develop his "gift," Gooch began attending her weekly circle, which consisted entirely of mediumistic individuals.

Sometimes Gooch and the other mediums would channel "higher guides." Other times they would hold what's called a "rescue circle," whereby they would channel the spirits of those who did not realize they were dead, their aim being to help them "move on." In *The Paranormal*, Gooch explains what it's like to be "possessed by one of these lost souls." It feels, he says, "as if another being 'materializes' or arises within one's body and pervades it… There is a very clear and definite sense of another person within you."

During one particularly memorable séance, a cave man materialized in the corner of the room. "It stood half in shadow, watching us, breathing heavily as if nervous," says Gooch. He later came to suspect that this figure – "which so very much impressed and haunted me both then and afterwards" – was a Neanderthal. Years later, in 1971, Gooch formulated the hybrid-origin theory, which basically posits that we – Homo sapiens –

are a hybrid cross between the two early species of man, Neanderthal and Cro-Magnon. His *Total Man* trilogy is an exploration of this hypothesis. On another occasion, soon after the presiding medium said they would experience "a wondrous radiance," Gooch and the others were illuminated by what appeared to be a bright light shining down from above.

Eventually, Peter allowed Gooch to have a session with his spirit guide, an alleged American Indian named Grey Hawk. While Peter was channeling Grey Hawk, his face and profile took on the features of a "storybook Indian." Grey Hawk gave Gooch a long lecture on "the nature of spirit," which Gooch found moving and poetic, though also empty and unsatisfying. As the reader may recall, Gooch says he finds many talks by spirit guides, as well as the books they have dictated, "a kind of intellectual candy-floss."

Gooch believes that Grey Hawk and other so-called discarnate entities are nothing more than creations of the unconscious minds of the mediums who channel them. Not surprisingly, he gives the "spirit hypothesis" very little consideration. He does state, however, that it would be arrogant to rule out the possibility that some channeled entities are indeed the spirits of the dead.

As an example of how channeled information, as a general rule, leaves much to be desired, Gooch mentions the numerous Seth books that have been written through Jane Roberts. Some of the other "personalities" that have supposedly been channeled by Roberts include the eminent psychologists William James and C.G. Jung, the latter of whom, as Gooch points out, must have lost the plot as a result of "crossing over."

To show just how barmy Jung has become, Gooch gives an example of one of his speeches taken from Robert's book *Psychic Politics*. Here is an excerpt: "Numbers have an emotional equivalent, in that their symbols arose from the libido that always identifies itself with the number 1, and feels all other numbers originating out of itself. The libido knows itself as God, and therefore all fractions fly out of the self structure of its own reality." Says Gooch: "If this is really Jung, speaking from the other side, then he has gone bananas."

As explained in his book *The Paranormal*, Gooch not only developed mediumistic powers, he also developed the ability to write automatically. "After only one or two attempts my hand began to write vigorously and fluently," he explains. To be successful in this endeavor, he says, you must be totally relaxed and in an environment free of distractions, paying as little attention to your "writing hand" as possible.

After much experimentation with automatic writing, Gooch reached the conclusion that his unconscious mind was producing the results. The types of "personalities" that expressed themselves on paper were many and varied, he says. He describes some of their comments as "solemn and soulful." Others, he says, were "naughty remarks of the 'impish spirit'. And occasionally the cursing and filth of the true demon or devil." Gooch soon discovered that, simply by using mental commands, he was able to alter the tone and style of the material he wrote automatically. This process, he insists, was purely mental, in that no amount of deliberate, physical force was used. "I could also lead the conversation in any direction I chose," he explains. "I could easily catch out the communicant by causing him or her to contradict something said earlier."

Gooch's views and experiences are certainly very compelling, while some of the evidence he presents in support of the unconscious mind theory is worth taking into consideration. The main problem with his argument, however, is that it doesn't take into account that most of the spirits who communicate through mediums are of an imperfect nature and are given to lying and deceiving, and this includes such ostensibly wise and learned beings as Seth. No wonder his friend's American Indian "spirit guide" spoke a load of hogwash, or, as he put it, "intellectual candy floss."

One of Gooch's main arguments against the spirit hypothesis is that "the alleged spirits never tell us anything that is not already known to living persons on this planet..." This, I have to admit, is a very good point. One theory to explain this – which we've already touched on – is that lower astral entities are able to read the minds of the living, stealing their ideas and memories and claiming them as their own; for it would appear that many such beings possess no real identity and are therefore required to fabricate one. They are merely shadows or fragments of their former selves. They exist, yet they do not exist – and this pains them terribly. Aviva Neumann's channeled "spirit guides" were obviously of this nature.

Unlike Gooch, I'm of the opinion that some spirit communications contain valuable, intelligent, and original information. The best example I can think of is *The Spirits' Book*, which, as I explained, contains scientific information that was not already known to persons living on the planet in 1857, the year it was published. Another notable example is the work of the late Brazilian Spiritist medium Chico Xavier, who wrote more than 400 books automatically, some of them bestsellers. I will present more information on Xavier and his work in the next chapter.

As for Gooch's experiences with automatic writing, whereby he was able to lead the conversation in any direction he choose, it's quite possible that he was "channeling" trickster entities, and that these entities were influencing his mind, causing him to think that he himself was creating the material that was written. Or maybe his mind did play a role, either small or large, in shaping or creating the material. Even if the latter were true, it doesn't change the fact that spirits may have influenced his mind to some extent. Mediumship is an imperfect process. The information that comes through a medium is never entirely "clean" in the sense that the medium's mind influences and colors it to some degree.

One could compare a medium to an electrical inverter that changes alternating current (AC) to direct current (DC). AC electricity is represented on a graph as a wave, because it reverses its direction or polarity at regularly recurring intervals. DC electricity, on the other hand, being a steady flow of charge in one direction, is represented on a graph as a straight line. DC, of course, has a frequency of zero, while the frequency of AC varies according to the rate at which the polarity changes – that is, the number of forwards-backwards cycles per second. Solar panels generate DC electricity of around 12 volts. In household solar power systems, this electricity is stored in batteries. So as to power common household appliances – almost all of which use AC – an inverter is used to convert the DC power from the batteries into AC power.

Spirits exist in a totally different realm – or frequency – to us. Let's call it the "DC realm." And let's call our realm the "AC realm." According to our analogy, the medium would be the inverter, who, shall we say, has a foot in both realms – the AC and the DC – and who, moreover, converts the "spirit's DC frequency" into something we can understand – "human AC frequency." But here's the catch – inverters or mediums are not totally efficient, efficiency being a measure of *how well* the conversion process occurs. For inverters, the average is around 90%. Nor, by comparison, are mediums 100% "efficient" because, as I said, their minds color and distort the information that comes through them from the spirit realm. The degree to which this happens depends on the competency of the medium.

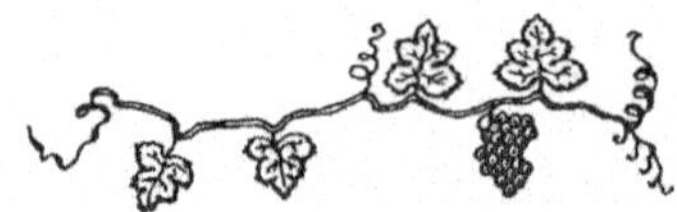

In the first chapter of *The Origins of Psychic Phenomena*, "Incubi and Succubi in Suburbia," Gooch describes the case of a former Metropolitan Police

Officer named Martyn Pryer, who at the age of forty-one began experimenting with hypnagogic imagery and found himself confronted by beings from the spirit realm. (Or, according to Gooch's interpretation of the matter, being in the hypnagogic state enabled Martin's conscious mind to encounter his unconscious mind.) Martin describes the process by which he was able to achieve this state: "On going to bed I would place a folded handkerchief over my eyes to keep out any residual light, and then physically relax. I would allow myself to drift down towards sleep and then try to hold myself just barely awake."

From then on, Martyn became a disturbed and restless sleeper, and would sometimes wake up in the middle of the night bathed in sweat. He also began to talk in his sleep. "And, once, during a vivid dream, I made an eerie, high-pitched whining. I was aware that I was doing it, but knew I could not stop till the dream was over." Disturbed by the noise, his wife would often go downstairs to sleep on the settee. After a mere three weeks, Martyn's hypnagogic experiments began to yield some interesting results. While in this state, he would sometimes hear knocking and thumping sounds, "quite different from house-settling noises or water pipes." He began to hear voices, too, and also conversations going on around him. One time he heard a nasty female voice cackle in his ear. On another occasion, he was addressed by a male voice, to which he replied.

Martyn's hypnagogic experiments became a little more daring when he tried to induce OBEs. He even attempted the "Kundalini effect." The results of these experiments varied. One night, while lying on his back, "relaxing and hypnagoging," Martyn felt something tug on his hair. A few nights later, while attempting to get to sleep, he heard a loud "whoosh" sound and was "seized from behind by a man-like entity." Martyn could not move. "It pinioned my legs with its legs, and my arms with its arms, and began breathing heavily in my ear." Martyn was able to "taste" the mind of his attacker – "this creature" – whom he felt to be "primitive, wanton, unprincipled, uncivilized – the opposite to all that is normally regarded as noble and good...It was Satan on my back."

Martyn describes what happened next: "Somehow a visionary experience now became entwined in the situation. I knew that I was still in bed (though that knowledge was very remote), but I was also standing in a very dark room – and in full possession of my normal faculties. I knew that there was a light switch just outside the room, and I managed to stagger across the room with the 'thing' clinging like a limpet on my back. I reached through the doorway for the light switch, only to find that this was hidden under a mass of trailing wires and cables. Scrabbling around through the wires, I finally got to the switch. But before I could press it, as I was about to do, I was released. I did not wake up. I had been awake all the time. But with a 'pop' the scene around me changed from the dark room to my bedroom."

Curious to see what would happen, Martyn continued with his hypnagogic experiments. The experiences he describes in Gooch's book are clearly SP episodes, though, apparently having no knowledge of the SP phenomenon at the time he wrote the book, Gooch refers to them as "incubi and succubi encounters."

Much like the episode described earlier, in which a "visionary experience" "became entwined in the situation," Martin, after practicing hypnagogy for a while, lay down on his side to go to sleep and suddenly found himself in total darkness. "I was fully awake and conscious – but I sensed that I was somehow in a different room…I made my way over to where I sensed there was a window. Outside was a girl…whom I had once courted in my youth. I asked: 'What are you doing here, Christine?' She replied: 'You sent for me.' I reached out and felt her face. I could really feel it. It was solid to my touch."

Suddenly, upon being seized from behind, Martyn was "knocked" into a different state of consciousness, in which he felt as though he were fully awake. Unable to move a muscle, he could sense that he was lying in bed and could feel an entity clasping him from behind. It was, he could tell, anthropomorphic and distinctly female. "It molded itself to my back and nuzzled the left side of the back of my neck." Instead of fighting the experience, as he had done previously, Martyn waited to see what would happen next. "It seemed to me that the entity was displaying an intention – a desire that was entirely its own, and a kind of nasty intelligence. It seemed, obviously, to want to make love to me, in a crude and violent manner." The presence of the entity soon faded, and Martyn eventually fell asleep.

In addition to Martyn's encounters, Gooch describes the "incubus" experiences of a female actor named Sandy, who while lying in bed one night felt an enormous pressure bearing down on her, as though a man were lying on top of her. As the "presence" began making gentle rhythmic motions, Sandy felt pressure on her vagina. She was in two minds about the prospect of giving herself to the presence. She began to struggle as the pressure increased and became painful. She felt another presence – this one extremely evil – dragging her down through the mattress. With great effort, she managed to haul herself free. She then woke up. Examining herself in the mirror, Sandy noticed that her mouth was rimmed with streaks of dried blood, and that her mouth was full of black blood. A medical examination revealed that her mouth and throat had not been injured, nor was there any sign of a nosebleed.

In the same book, Gooch describes several of his own "succubus" encounters, one of which occurred in his mid-twenties, when he was developing as a trance medium. While lying in bed on a Saturday morning, reluctant to get up, Gooch felt a "hand" press down on his pillow. He kept his eyes closed until the presence had departed. Gooch says he was "thrilled" by the experience, if not a little startled by it. In contrast to Martyn's and Sandy's encounters, he describes his own as "extremely pleasant."

His next "succubus" experience occurred about twenty years later, when, lying in bed in the early hours of the morning, he became aware of a "person" lying next to him, whom he could sense was female. She shifted closer towards him, pressing her body against his. Gooch quickly realized that she was a "psychic entity" and not a real person. He felt, more specifically, that she was "a composite of various girls I had once known, including my ex-wife, but with other elements not drawn from my memories in any sense." She was, he believes, a product of his unconscious mind.

Overcome by excitement, for it was clear that the entity wished to have sex with him, Gooch woke up. On another occasion, the entity appeared again, and this time they actually made love. Like a true gentlemen, Gooch refuses to comment on the intimate details of their lovemaking, though he does mention that the experience was "totally satisfying." He even goes as far as to say that "spirit sex" (my term, not his) "is actually more satisfying than with a real woman, because in the paranormal encounter archetypal elements are both involved and invoked…" He adds: "I am more than happy to settle for a relationship with a succubus, and the world of real women…can go whistle."

I can understand where Gooch is coming from with this last comment (no offence to real females), but I do have my suspicions as to whether or not "spirit sex" is entirely wholesome. According to American paranormal researcher Brad Steiger, consensual sex with a discarnate entity "is one of the most dangerous things a human can do – ultimately courting possession." I feel that Steiger may be right. Fisher, remember, was sexually involved with Filipa, and he ended up hurling himself off a cliff. Were I to encounter a succubus these days, I would most likely resist the temptation.

Interestingly, Gooch's view of the entity, as being a product of his unconscious mind rather than a spirit, is extremely contradictory. He mentions, for instance, that it was "essentially its own independent self…its own creature, but seemed, as it were, to be using part of my own experience in order to present itself to me." Reading these words, one gets the impression that Gooch had serious doubts as to the exact nature of the entity. Assuming the entity was a spirit – which in my opinion it probably was – and bearing in mind that spirits are masters of manipulation, able to appear in various forms, it makes sense that the entity used, in Gooch's words, "part of my own experience in order to present itself to me." Did I not explain earlier that succubi and incubi, according to legend, are able to alter their form so as to appear more sexually appealing to those whom they wish to seduce?

In an article entitled "Vampires: Do They Exist?" Wilson makes a valuable point in opposition to the "unconscious mind" interpretation of Gooch's "succubus" experiences. "It seems obvious," he says, "that he arrived at that conclusion because his 'succubus' seemed to be a blend of previous girlfriends. But according to the 'earth-bound spirit' hypothesis, we would assume that the entity simply put these ideas into his mind – that is, into his imagination." Wilson adds: "We also note that these 'psychic invasions' occurred when all three subjects – Gooch, Martyn Pryer, and Sandy – were either asleep or hovering between sleep and waking, *and therefore in a trance condition akin to mediumship*" (my emphasis).

Gooch, like Martyn, underwent his "succubus" experiences while in a state of semi-consciousness between wakefulness and sleep. In Gooch's case it was the hypnopompic state, and in Martyn's the hypnagogic. They are, as I've said, basically the same state of consciousness – the same "frequency," if you will. Both men enjoyed experimenting with altered states. They, like the shaman, were able to train their minds in such a way as to sustain the duration of the hypnagogic and hypnopompic states, but with varying results.

A little about shamanism needs to be mentioned at this juncture, because the ability to control one's state of consciousness, and indeed the ability to enter and sustain a trance state, is such a fundamental part of the shamanic process. Some of the consciousness-altering techniques employed by shamans include beating a drum to a certain frequency (usually of around four to seven cycles per second); singing repetitive and monotonous "power songs"; and, of course, taking psychoactive substances, such as Ayahuasca (which contains the hallucinogenic alkaloid DMT), or Psilocybin mushrooms. All of these methods allow the shaman to enter what the anthropologist Michael Harner calls a "shamanic state of consciousness" (SSC).

According to Philip Gardiner and Gary Osborne in their book *The Shining Ones*, the ancient shamans viewed consciousness as a traveling sine wave, with the "negative" half of the cycle representing the period during which we are asleep, and the "positive" half of the cycle representing the period during which we are awake. If one were to picture this in one's mind, the line passing straight through the middle of the graph would represent the null line or timeline, and one peak and one trough would equal one cycle – which, as we know, is roughly a twenty-four hour period. This is called a circadian rhythm, or the sleep-wake cycle.

The sleep-wake cycle not only consists of a positive (wakefulness) phase and a negative (asleep) phase but also a neutral (transliminal) phase. (The word "transliminal" comes from the Latin, for "crossing the boundary" or "threshold.") These neutral phases – or nodes – are those points on the graph where the opposites, or two halves of a cycle, are briefly united. And these, of course, would represent the hypnopompic and hypnagogic states. During a complete cycle, you cross the hypnagogic phase before falling asleep, and, before waking up, you cross the hypnopompic phase. Most people, of course, are totally unconscious during these phases – the SP sufferer and the shaman being two exceptions. "The neutral point in the cycle," explains Gardiner and Osborne, "is where the opposites meet and are briefly unified – neutralized as separate phenomena. Therefore, for the ancient shaman, this formed a correspondence with the sexual union of male and female which produces that 'creative spark.'"

Not only can the sleep-wake cycle be represented as a traveling sine wave, says Gardiner and Osborne, but so too can our own state of consciousness, which cycles or oscillates many times a second, "and in every instant we fluctuate momentarily between conscious and subconscious, with the unconscious 'zero node' crossed twice every cycle." To comprehend this better, think of the "positive" half of the cycle as representing the conscious self, which is objective and male, and the "negative" half of the cycle as representing the subconscious, which is subjective and female. The neutral points in the cycle represent the unconscious. "If we become conscious at these points," adds Gardiner and Osborne, "as in the hypnagogic state, then everything collapses into the centre or superconscious." It could be said, then, that the SP state allows one access to a superconscious level of mind.

Various techniques are employed by the shaman to enter a trance state, several of which I've already mentioned, such as beating a drum. There is another method, too, and it's one that Martyn Pryer was obviously well aware of. What one has to do is to try and remain awake and aware at the point of going to sleep, which, as we know, enables one to enter the hypnagogic state. Shamans regard the hypnagogic state as a "gateway" or "portal" to other realms, one of them being the underworld. "In these 'other worlds' or 'other-dimensional realms,'" writes Osborne and Gardiner, "the shaman encountered all kinds of creature, even human-animal hybrids…He also 'met' and interacted with dead people, friends, relatives and ancestors who would sometimes pass on important information which he could use to his benefit, *although some would try to trick him and even do him harm* [my emphasis]. We can see why he believed that this realm was the underworld, the world of the dead…"

Speaking of shamanic journeys to the underworld, the hypnagogic experiences of Martyn Pryer spring to mind. These experiences, he insists, felt very real indeed and could not have been dreams – at least not regular dreams. Were they, then, lucid dreams? Or perhaps OBEs? My feeling is that they were lucid dreams (LDs), keeping in mind that these experiences, in the words of Sevilla, a lucid dreamer himself, "are usually vivid, almost always in color (for me) and rich in detail."

Included in *Wrestling with Ghosts* is an article by Lucy Gillis – producer and co-editor of *The Lucid Dreaming Exchange* journal and website – in which she examines the relationship between SP, LDs, and OBEs. Gillis has experienced all three phenomena herself, and she makes a distinction between the second and third, explaining that OBEs are "not just vivid dreams." The SP state, she says, is not only a "gateway" to the out-of-body state but to lucid dreaming as well because "the sleep paralysis 'sufferer' is experiencing what the lucid dreamer strives for: awareness during sleep." One can use the SP state to one's advantage, she says, by learning to carry one's awareness into the dream state.

Gillis makes it clear that although LDs and OBEs are separate phenomena, they're not that far removed, while it's possible for some advanced dreamers such as herself to shift voluntarily from one to the other. You could be having a LD, for example, and then suddenly decide to move into an out-of-body state. Not all researchers agree, by the way, that there are any significant differences between LDs and OBEs, viewing them instead as two aspects of the same underlying experience.

In addition to Gillis, another researcher who draws a distinction between the two phenomena is British psychologist, author and paranormal skeptic Susan Blackmore. One of the major differences she lists is that most OBEs occur during waking, while most LDs occur during REM sleep. "This division is obscured by the fact that some experiences resembling OBEs occur in sleep," she explains. "Some researchers count these as OBEs while others do not." Another difference she mentions is that OBEs – "perhaps only by convention or definition" – take place in what appears to be the physical world, while LDs can occur in any imagined setting.

Most of us know that a LD is a dream in which one is aware that one is dreaming while the dream is in progress. Extremely real and vivid, LDs are such that it's possible to exert conscious control over the events that occur in the dream, as well as other aspects of the dream. In addition, the dreamer is able to perform various physical feats that would otherwise be impossible. One can float, glide, fly, hover, jump great distances – the examples are endless. Sevilla mentions that one can sometimes hear, and even compose, music while in the "LD universe." It possesses, he says, "a great degree of richness and surrealism, beyond what real music would sound like (ethereal)."

Just as there are degrees of vividness when it comes to regular dreams, so there are degrees of lucidity when it comes to LDs. Very few of us have ever had a LD of extremely high degree. Children have them more often than adults, and, as I made clear, SP sufferers are more likely to have them than non-SP sufferers. Gooch calls the "LD universe" the "inner alternative world of the mind," and in *The Origins of Psychic Phenomena* he explains what it's like to journey to such a place. His means of entering the "inner world," he explains, is through the hypnopompic state. "I become aware that I am almost awake and mentally decline to wake further." The experiences Gooch describes are reminiscent of shamanic journeys to the underworld.

While in a trance state (commonly of the hypnagogic kind) the shaman will slip into another reality, entering an "imaginary" hole in the earth and eventually reaching the underworld. "The entrance among California Indian shamans, for example, frequently was a spring, especially a hot one," writes Harner in *The Way of the Shaman*. "Shamans were reputed to travel hundreds of miles underground, entering one hot spring and coming out at another." The reasons for undertaking such a journey are many. Sometimes the shaman's aim is to bring back important knowledge, or to heal a patient, by recovering the patient's "guardian power animal," making sure it's brought back safely, and is restored to them.

Harner, who has not only studied shamanism as an anthropologist but is also an authentic shaman himself, having been taught by both the Shuar (Jivaro) and Conibo tribes of the Amazon, comments on the SSC as though it is identical to the lucid dreaming state. The shaman's "experiences are like dreams, but waking ones that feel real and in which he can control his actions and direct his adventures. While in the SSC, he is often amazed by the reality of that which is presented. He gains access to a whole new, and yet familiarly ancient universe that provides him with profound information about the meaning of his own life and death and his place within the totality of all existence."

As for Gooch's "trips to the inner universe" – the inner universe, in his view, being his own unconscious mind – they usually commence, he says, with a feeling of movement. "The movement appears wholly real and literal. I may dive backwards, head first, through the pillow and down through the floor and soon am in rapid free fall...Then I may land, with a little bump...on the floor of a cellar with a passageway leading off. When I get up and go through the door, or the passage, I am in the magic world." This description, by the way, is consistent with typical shamanic journeys to the underworld, the passage or tunnel through which one slides or falls often appearing as a long, ribbed tube, the end of which is flooded by light, like one would find at the entrance of a cave. One emerges through this entrance – or exit, if you like – into another landscape, this being the underworld, which might be marked by trees, mountains, and streams, and might, also, feature a beautiful blue sky.

Gooch continues with his description of the "inner universe": "I might be running through a beautiful countryside, delighting in the air, the sunshine, and the sights and sounds of nature. Then perhaps I come to, or start off in, a town. Here the architecture is of amazing beauty and variety. Yet there is prosaic life too. There will be streets of shops and cafes, with many people in them. It is all full of interest, all totally new and unexpected... Yet the best part of all is the triumphant feeling of being there, of having escaped from all the cares and limitations of the daily human grind, of being in my own personal wonderland where all is possible, and where the imagination can never be exhausted. I talk to the people. I may meet a girl, and with luck, go to bed with her. The sex is not just as good as, but better than that obtained in the real world, because one's own personal archetypal wishes and fantasies may be, and often are, lived out."

Unlike the shaman who ascribes some objectivity to his journeys to the underworld, Gooch is of the opinion that these experiences lie solely with the unconscious mind. And indeed he may be partially right, for it cannot be doubted that we underestimate the mind's potential, that we possess "unknown powers," that the human imagination is a very potent thing, and that, in a sense, the unconscious mind is another universe in itself, of which most of us have barely scraped the surface. The clinical psychologist Wilson Van Dusen, whose work we will explore later on, likens the mind to a vast castle, filled with relics, countless rooms, dungeons, and artifacts. We spend our lives "locked up in such a mind-castle," he says, "yet we have explored little. Many know little more than a sitting room in the east wing and assume this is the whole."

CHAPTER 10

Chico Xavier: The Pope Of Spiritism

Not only does June 30, 2002, mark the winning of the World Cup for Brazil, it also marks the death of one of the country's most successful and prolific authors, who, believe it or not, was also a Spiritist medium, having written all of his books automatically – more than four hundred – some of which were bestsellers. His name was Francisco de Paula Candido Xavier, better known as Chico Xavier. A true Christian Spiritist who gave every cent he earned to the poor and whose entire life was dedicated to helping others, Xavier will forever be remembered for the charity and spiritual upliftment he brought to the lives of many.

One of nine children, Xavier was born on April 2, 1910, in the small town of Pedro Leopoldo, located in the south-eastern state of Minas Gerais. His mother died when he was five years old, so a godmother adopted Xavier. That same year, he apparently saw his mother's ghost and from then on began to experience spirit phenomena on a frequent basis, hearing voices and sensing unseen presences. Thinking he was under the influence of the devil, his godmother, a mean and abusive woman, used to beat him several times a day, and oftentimes Xavier would hide in the backyard. As penance, the local priest ordered him to say a thousand Ave Marias and to walk around with a 15kg stone on his head.

One day, while at primary school, Xavier and his classmates were asked to write an essay on the history of Brazil as part of a state government run competition. While seated at his desk, wondering what to put down on paper, Xavier was approached by a man, whom only he could see. The man started talking, as though dictating what to write, beginning with the words: "Brazil, discovered by Pedro Alvares Cabral, may be compared to the most precious diamond in the world which was soon to be set in the Crown of Portugal..." The young Xavier copied it all down, winning an honorable mention in the competition. His classmates, not to mention his teacher, were greatly surprised by his new "talent." They were more surprised still when he gave all the credit to a spirit.

As proof that his essay had indeed been dictated by a spirit, Xavier was asked to write another one, this time on the topic of "sand" – a topic randomly chosen by one of his fellow students, much to the amusement of the rest of the class. Xavier did not disappoint. He went straight to the blackboard, picked up a piece of chalk, and began writing: "My sons, creation is not mocked. A grain of sand is almost nothing, yet it appears as a tiny star reflecting the son of God…" It's fair to assume that there must have been a few stunned faces in the classroom that day. The teacher, a catholic, forbade the students to discuss such matters as unseen voices ever again, later telling Xavier to pray for spiritual guidance.

At the age of eleven, while still at school, Xavier was required to start working to support himself financially. His first job was at a textile plant, where he stayed for four years. He left school at age thirteen, having completed primary level – which, points out Playfair in his book *The Flying Cow*, "was scarcely adequate training for a boy who was to become the country's most prolific author." Until his retirement in 1961 at the age of about fifty, Xavier held a number of modest jobs. He worked as a kitchen hand, a shop assistant, and lastly as a fingerprint expert with the Ministry of Agriculture, where he was employed for some thirty years.

Xavier's career as a practicing medium began in 1927, after one of his sisters allegedly went insane. She had been taken to a local healing medium, diagnosed as a victim of "spirit possession," and promptly cured. Everyone who had witnessed her remarkable recovery was greatly impressed, especially the Xavier family who renounced Christianity right then and there and became Spiritists. Also amazed by the extraordinary incident, the healing medium's wife, Carmen Peracio, decided to found a small evangelical Spiritist center, which Xavier began attending. During one session held in 1927, Mrs. Peracio heard a voice instructing her to hand Xavier a pencil and some paper, which she did. A moment later, Xavier handed her a seventeen-page message of spiritual guidance, which he had written automatically in a state of trance. (The Spiritists call automatic writing "psychography," and one who practices psychography, a "psychographic" medium.)

During another session, Mrs. Peracio had a vision of a man dressed in priest's robes who introduced himself as "Emmanuel." The man, who had a brilliant aura, told her he was Xavier's spiritual friend. About four years later, in 1931, Xavier also "met" Emmanuel, whom he came to believe was his chief spirit guide. In previous incarnations Emmanuel is said to have been both the Roman senator Publius Lentulus and the Portuguese Jesuit priest Manuel de Nobrega. Through Xavier, Emmanuel would go on to write a series of bestselling, historic novels.

In another significant vision, Mrs. Peracio saw a shower of books fall around Xavier's head. This, she believed, was a sign that he had an important spiritual mission to fulfill. When she described the vision to Xavier, he misheard her, thinking she'd used the word *lirio* (lily) instead of *livro* (book). Thus he was left puzzled as to what it all meant. Why, he thought to himself, would a developing medium such as he be honored with a shower of flowers?

While still employed at the Ministry of Agriculture, Xavier wrote – or rather, fifty-six different discarnate poets wrote – a 421-page volume of poetry containing 256 poems entitled *Parnassus from Beyond the Tomb*. Written by the Keats and Byrons of the Portuguese language, this highly impressive and controversial book, published in 1932 by the Brazilian Spiritist Federation (FEB), became an immediate bestseller. According to Playfair, the book was still in print in 1975 and had sold, as of that date, some 40,000 copies. Presumably this figure is now much higher. The book contains poems by such distinguished Brazilian and Portuguese poets as Guerra Junqueiro, Antero de Quental, Augusto dos Anjos, Castro Avles, and many others; each poem is written in the author's own distinctive style.

Decades after it was published, the book was still causing a sensation in Brazil. That it was written by a twenty-one-year-old, half-literate fingerprint expert who hadn't even attended secondary school was simply too much for some people to swallow. Even more difficult to accept is that the poems in the book were the work of actual, discarnate poets. Nevertheless, few could deny that the poems were impressive.

The late Monteiro Lobato, one of Brazil's most influential authors and best known for his children's books, had nothing but praise for Xavier's book of poems from beyond the grave. "If the man produced all this on his own," he once commented, "then he can occupy as many chairs in the academy as he likes!"

But the most notable admirer, among the many Brazilian intellectuals and literary critics, was Humberto de Campos, a journalist and leading literary figure of his time. Having studied the poems carefully, Campos concluded: "I would fail the duty imposed upon me by my conscience if I did not confess that, making verses through the pen of Mr. Francisco Candido Xavier, the poets of whom he is the interpreter present the same characteristics of inspiration and expression that identified them on this planet. The themes broached are the same that preoccupied them when alive. The taste is the same. And the verse answers, as a rule, to the same musical rhythms..." It should be noted that Campos had a reputation for being a sharp-tongued critic and a difficult man to please.

Oddly enough, Campos died about two years after the publication of *Parnassus* and quickly become a member of Xavier's "team" of discarnate authors. Through Xavier he wrote a total of five books between 1937 and 1942, all of them highly praised. While producing these books, by the way, Xavier had been busy working on other projects as well. He wrote at an astonishing pace, three books a year on average. As of 1971, the discarnate Campos had written a total of twelve books, bringing his sales to 323,000 copies.

According to Campos's mother, Ana de Campos Veras, in an interview published in 1944, these books – with titles like *New Messages* (1940) and *Good Tidings* (1941), the latter of which concerned the teachings of Jesus – were indeed written in the exact same style as her son's. "I have no doubt in stating this," she added, "and there is no scientific explanation for the fact." As though the entire affair wasn't bizarre enough already, Campos's widow and his publishers decided to sue Xavier and his publishers; the reason being, they said, that if the books really were by Campos, then they were entitled to some author's rights and ought to be receiving royalties.

The lawsuit involved having to decide whether or not Campos had written the books in question from beyond the grave and therefore whether or not there is such thing as an afterlife. This, explains Pedro McGregor in his book *The Moon and Two Mountains*, "was an impossible task – to ask a terrestrial court to decided on the existence or otherwise, in fact, of the hereafter." But because Campos was officially dead and the dead have no rights, the judge dismissed the case. Due to all the publicity he received as a result of the affair, Xavier's books sold better than ever before.

In the first chapter of *The Flying Cow*, Playfair relates the time he met Xavier at a book signing in the Sao Paulo satellite town of Sao Bernardo do Compo in the 1970s. Almost a thousand people attended the event, all of whom were eager to meet – and have their books signed by – the great medium himself. When it came to his turn, says Playfair, "Chico greeted me as if there were nobody he wanted to meet more...signed three books for me and gave me two red roses and a warm handshake...Chico, I was assured, would not leave his post until everybody had been given an autograph, a handshake and a souvenir rose, even if this would take all night."

Playfair describes Xavier quite flatteringly as a "one-man welfare service" and an individual "of almost pathological modesty and humility," noting that he never sought fame, always put the needs of other's above his own, and refused to accept any payment for the sale of his books, instead spending the money – every cent of it – on food, clothing, and medical assistance for the poor. Had he wanted to, insists Playfair, Xavier could easily have become a millionaire – even if he had accepted only a very small percentage of the money generated from the sale of his books. Also, adds Playfair, had Xavier claimed that he alone, and not the various spirits, had written all of his books, he would have been recognized "as one of the most versatile literary geniuses of his time."

Xavier's books, all of which were published by Spiritist publishing houses, have been translated into several different languages, including English, Japanese, French, Esperanto, and Greek. So far, only three of his books are available in English; I own one, *In the Domain of Mediumship: Life in the Spiritual World* (1955). On the front cover of this attractive, well-produced book, Xavier's name is mentioned, as is the name of the spirit it was allegedly written by – Andre Luiz, apparently a former physician (thought to be the famous Oswaldo Cruz). Of all the spirits who wrote through Xavier, Luiz's work has sold the most. The first book to bear Luiz's name, a novel entitled *Nosso Lar* (*Our Home*), had sold more than 120,000 copies by 1975, becoming his all-time bestseller. According to a recent estimate, 25 million copies of Xavier's books have been sold.

If, as a number of skeptics have claimed, Xavier was a deceptive genius who wrote his books by normal human means, or, according to another theory, his subconscious mind was responsible, it still remains difficult to explain how he managed to write so prolifically, and in so many different styles and genres. His works include poetry, children's books, historical and contemporary novels, as well as treatises on religion, science, and philosophy. It cannot be denied, of course, that the world has seen some extremely versatile and prolific writers – take the late Isaac Asimov, for example, who wrote some 400 books, including works of science-fiction, popular science, mystery fiction, literary criticism, and so on. Impressive though this is, Asimov's work, compared to Xavier's, is extremely limited in scope. Though of course, as with anything of a paranormal nature, one could debate the authenticity of Xavier's alleged psychic ability till the cows come home.

A significant portion of Xavier's automatic writing took place during Spiritist sessions in full view of witnesses. On every occasion, Xavier would enter a trance state, his left hand resting over his weak eye (in which, from a young age, he was almost entirely blind, making it difficult for him to read). The many people who saw him write were amazed by the speed at which he was able to do so. One witness described his hand as moving "as if driven by a battery." Usually, while Xavier's hand was flying across the page, an assistant would sit nearby, keeping him supplied with paper.

"When I am writing automatically," Xavier once said, "I can see, hear, and feel the discarnate spirit who is working by means of my arm, and I have often registered the presence of the communicator without knowing anything about the subject matter on which he is writing." According to Xavier, the sensation he felt while writing the poems in *Parnassus* "was that a vigorous hand was propelling my own. Sometimes there seemed to be a non-material volume in front of me, where I read and copied them; while at other times it seemed more like somebody dictating them into my ears."

In what seems to have been a deliberate attempt to convince even the most stubborn skeptics of the reality of mediumship, Luiz wrote, through Xavier and another medium – a young physician named Waldo Vieira – a highly technical book entitled *Evolution in Two Worlds* (1959) on the functioning of both the physical and spiritual worlds. To produce this obscure, collaborative work, Xavier, while in Pedro Leopoldo, would write one chapter, while Vieira, living in a separate city 200 miles away, would write the next a few days later, without having any contact with the other, each taking turns as the medium.

The book, consisting of forty chapters, took a little over five months to complete, at which point Xavier was instructed by Emmanuel to contact Vieira so that they could put their halves of the manuscript together. Amazingly, the style of *Evolution* is consistent throughout. The book demonstrates, according to Playfair, "an immense knowledge of several sciences that no ordinary writer, even a qualified scientist, could have assembled without copious research and note-taking, and despite the wide education gap between the two writers, the unity of style is complete."

In 1958, Xavier suddenly walked out of his home without telling his neighbors where he was going and went to live in the city of Uberaba, Minas Gerais, located about 250 miles away. The only belongings he took with him were the clothes he was wearing. About twelve years later, when a reporter went to visit his previous home, they found everything untouched, exactly as Xavier had left it. Apparently, one of his suits was still hanging from a wardrobe door. The reason he decided to move, Xavier always insisted, was because he thought the climate of Uberaba, being more temperate to that of Pedro Leopoldo, would be of benefit to his health. The truth of the matter is, however, that Xavier's main reason for "skipping town" was due to an unpleasant incident concerning his nephew.

Perhaps out of jealousy or resentment, Xavier's nephew attempted to discredit his uncle and harm his reputation by announcing in public that

Xavier was a fraud and that all of his books were his own work. According to the nephew, Xavier possessed – and had always possessed – the impressive ability to imitate the literary styles of others. Not one shred of evidence existed to support this outlandish accusation, and it's fair to assume that the entire affair caused Xavier a great deal of sorrow, especially considering that a member of his own family was responsible. Rather than stay in Pedro Leopoldo and remain in conflict with his nephew, Xavier obivously thought it best to make a clean break. The nephew drank himself to death not long after making the accusation against Xavier.

At Uberaba, where he lived for the remainder of his life, Xavier helped transform a small Spiritist center into a large welfare organization. Named after the spirit Andre Luiz, the center provides food and clothing, such as shoes and blankets, to the poor people of the district. When Playfair visited the centre in the late 1970s, he noticed that some eight hundred bowls of soup were prepared and given to the hungry each day. People would come from all over Brazil to attend sessions at the center, as well as to receive from the spirits who communicated through Xavier, a personal message written on a piece of paper, usually in regards to a medical or spiritual problem.

A highly disciplined, dedicated, and energetic individual, Xavier rose each morning before seven, after about four hours sleep, and would spend most days typing up his manuscripts, replying to the hundreds of letters he received each day, visiting sick and needy people in the neighborhood, and attending Spiritist sessions. Interestingly, Xavier never married, remaining celibate his whole life. "I resisted the temptation of the flesh, and it was not easy," he once commented. "I didn't come to this life to get married. My commitment is with channeling and my spiritual family is already a large one."

Xavier was twice nominated for the Nobel Peace Prize: in 1981 and 1982. He died in 2002, age 92, of heart failure. That he passed away on the same day that the Brazilian soccer team won its fifth World Cup was apparently no coincidence. Xavier prophesized that his death would occur on a day of national celebration so as to lessen the grief of those who would miss him. Islamic, Jewish, and Christian religious leaders all paid tribute to Brazil's most respected medium, as did the country's president at the time, Fernando Henrique Cardoso. "To find the way to salvation," wrote the famous Brazilian doctor and playwright Pedro Bloch, "humanity needs a few million Chico Xaviers, even if they do not write a single message. For Chico Xavier himself is already a message…"

What Xavier achieved as a psychographic medium is particularly impressive when one considers that most channeled material is of a very low standard and has a limited appeal. To repeat a humorous quote from D. Scott Rogo's *The Infinite Boundary*: "I find that most channeled discourses possess the spiritual and philosophical sophistication of a Dick-and-Jane book." Indeed, Rogo's critical opinion seems to ring true of most channeled works, such as those written through Jane Roberts by the personality known as Seth, for example, or the extremely dull novels and poetry of the alleged spirit Patience Worth, channeled by the American housewife Pearl Curran. Xavier's material, on the other hand, is compelling and rich; in no way is it vague or without substance. Referring to his novels, Playfair points out that their plots "are as carefully structured as those of any others writer's" and that every one of his major works "shows evidence of sound literary craftsmanship, narrative skill being matched by vivid delineation of any kind of character."

Xavier's books can be divided into four major categories – literature, history, Spiritist doctrine, and science. The literature section is by far the most popular. Xavier's all time bestseller, the aforementioned *Nosso Lar* (*Our Home*), written by the spirit Andre Luiz, is a fascinating and absorbing work of fiction, containing much wisdom. In the first chapter of this apparently semi-autobiographical story, the protagonist, Luiz, finds himself in the lower zones of the spirit realm, having died of a severe intestinal occlusion, a condition brought about by drinking and eating to excess. The lower zones, the book explains, "are the shadowy regions where excessively self-centered souls or those with a guilt ridden conscience find themselves after death."

Examining his conscience, Luiz begins to realize that he lived a largely selfish and unproductive life. "I had lived on Earth, enjoyed its benefits, reaped the good things of life," he says, "and yet never contributed anything towards the repayment of my heavy debt. I had completely ignored my parent's generosity and sacrifices, just as I had ignored those of my wife and children. I had selfishly kept my family only to myself. I had been given a happy home, and had closed my doors to those seeking help. I had delighted in the joys of my family circle, yet never shared that precious gift with my greater human family. I had neglected to undertake even the most elementary duties of fraternal solidarity."

Luiz is eventually "rescued" from the lower zones by a group of kind souls and taken to a transit city called Our Home. The city is a very real place, with a government, public transportation system, and even houses and cinemas. The citizens of Our Home put themselves to work, so as to keep the city running, while they either prepare to be reborn on earth, or to ascend to a higher plane. In an effort to amend his sins, and give something back to the larger spiritual community, Luiz procures a job as a nurse in the Chambers of Rectification – a kind of hospital, where troubled and tormented souls who have been rescued from the lower zones spend time recovering. Feeling overly sorry for the patients, Luiz is told by one of the doctors to bear in mind "that their suffering is of their own doing. Man's life is always centered wherever his heart is."

In the Domain of Mediumship (1955) is another fascinating book in the Our Home series, of which there are fifteen altogether. Written in the first-person, this entertaining and accessible book, which is more a work of "spiritual science" than a novel, follows the protagonist and his friend Hilario as they journey around the physical plane, learning about the ins and outs of mediumship – not from our perspective, but from that of a spirit. Their instructor, Aulus, takes them to a Spiritist center, among other places, where they are gives the opportunity to witness mediumship in action.

At one Spiritist session, the protagonist sees a group of ill and disturbed spirits gathered around the incarnate mediums, "like moths instinctively drawn to a great light," many of whom desire to communicate with loved ones they've left behind and need help "moving on." So as to receive counseling, some of the sick spirits are given the opportunity to temporarily "possess" the body of one of the mediums and thus communicate through them. This, as we know, is called full trance mediumship.

Aulus explains how it works: "Although he uses Eugina's [the medium's] forces, the sick spirit is controlled by her nervous magnetic energy, through which our sister is informed of the words he intends to say. He has taken temporary possession of our sister's vocal cords and senses, thereby managing to discern, listen and reason with a certain amount of equilibrium through her energies. Eugenia, however, firmly controls the reigns of her will, operating as if she were a benevolent nurse helping a patient by agreeing with his requests. Yet she sets a limit on his desires because, conscious of the intentions of the unfortunate companion to whom she lends her physical body, she reserves the right to correct any undesirable conduct."

Second in popularity to Luiz's books are those written by Emmanuel, Xavier's chief spirit guide. His early works, which were produced while Xavier was still working fulltime, include a number of lengthy historic novels, one of which is more than 500 pages long and took eight months to put down on paper. Each novel contain a wealth of detailed information about the civilization in which it is set and is written from the perspective of one who was there at the time. Emmanuel's first novel, *Two Thousand Years Ago*, tells the story of Emperor Tiberius's envoy to Palestine. This book, like Emmanuel's other works of fiction, is filled with detailed descriptions of sex – which, given the fact that Xavier was celibate and most likely a virgin, are unlikely to have come from his own imagination. According to McGregor, *Two Thousand Years Ago* "has all the ingredients of the great novel and the best-seller..."

Emmanuel has also written, through Xavier, a number of books on Spiritist doctrine, such as *On the Path of Light*, an examination of history as perceived by those beyond the physical world. According to the book, humanity is currently on the brink of a cataclysm, after which will follow an age of peace and enlightenment. In Emmanuel's own words, the earth "is in a twilight which will be followed by a profound night, and the twenty-first century will witness the outcome of these dreadful events." We are also reaching the end of a cycle of evolution, says Emmanuel, "and the more the scientists advance, the more will they be aware of the subjective realities in universal phenomena."

In light of these dramatic predictions, it's reassuring to realize that, unlike so many other well-known spirit guides or highly evolved entities, Emmanuel never claimed to be infallible, as evidenced by a warning he once gave Xavier: "If one day I provide you with counsel that is not in conformity with Jesus and Kardec, stay with them and forget me." Emmanuel also stressed the point that spirits such as himself cannot solve all of humanities problems, or take over our destinies; the difficulties that we undergo are a necessary part of our evolution.

CHAPTER 11

Dion Fortune On Psychic Attack

I woke from a troubled sleep, but remained in a twilight state, as if under a spell. There was a growing chill in the air, or in my mind. I saw a soft glow and a menacing shape which brooded evil and which I thought I recognized. I knew I was in danger, but the peril was not on the physical plane. – G.R.S Mead (from *The Haunted Mind* by Nandor Fodor)

In his book *Mysteries*, Colin Wilson tells the intriguing story of the time his friend Bill Slater, former head of BBC Television drama, underwent a "psychic attack." One evening in the early 1950s, Slater, then a drama student, attended a party that eventually turned into a séance with a Ouija board. A Ouija board features letters, numbers, and other signs around its edge, and is used to communicate with spirits. A moveable pointer – sometimes a small, upturned glass – is located in the middle of the board, upon which the participants in the séance will place their index fingers ever so gently. Working through the participants, their mediumistic capacity combined, the communicating spirit is able to influence the movement of the pointer and thus spell out its answers. The pointer appears to move of its own accord.

Slater saw the glass move rapidly from letter to letter as it spelled out the answers to various questions. Though he found the phenomenon interesting, he thought it was nothing more than a party game. When he made some facetious remarks, the communicator became angry and resentful, and, when asked if it would like anyone to leave, the glass shot straight towards Slater. Bored with the "game" anyway, Slater was more than happy to withdraw, and off he went to flirt with an attractive girl. He returned home in the early hours of the morning, accompanied by a fellow drama student. After talking for a while they went to bed.

Two hours later, Slater had a frightening experience, an account of which he detailed in a letter to Wilson: "I found myself half-awake, knowing there was some kind of presence massing itself on my chest; it was, to my certain knowledge, making every effort to take over my mind and body. It cost me considerable will-power to concentrate all my faculties to push the thing away, and for what seemed like twenty minutes this spiritual tussle went on between this awful presence and myself. Needless to say, although before going to bed I had felt perfectly happy and at ease with a very good friend, in a flat I knew well, I was now absolutely terrified – I have never known such fear since. I was finally able to call my friend's name; he woke up, put on the light, and was astonished to find me well-nigh a gibbering idiot. I have never since had any psychic experience."

The literature on paranormal phenomena contains numerous descriptions of SP attacks, much like Slater's, that either took place while the victim was staying in a haunted house, directly after a "curse" had been placed on the victim, or when the victim was dabbling in spirit communications, such as with the use of a Ouija board. Either we choose to accept the theory that SP attacks occur on a largely random basis and are nothing more than a neurological glitch, or we examine the evidence closely, look for patterns, and come to realize that at least some SP attacks, such as Slater's, are directly related to the influence of spirits. A skeptic would declare that Slater's SP experience had nothing to do with the séance he attended, that the two incidents are in no way linked. All the evidence presented so far clearly indicates otherwise, however.

Further evidence that some SP attacks are caused by the influence of spirits can be found in a case reported by the Jungian psychoanalyst Mary Williams and published in the extremely respectable *Journal of Analytical Psychology*. The case is also mentioned in Gooch's *The Origins of Psychic Phenomena*. It concerns one of William's patients, a handsome man of thirty-two named Roger, whose psychic troubles began when he started attending séances. In one session, everyone present witnessed a "violet light," and Roger, who was accompanied by his girlfriend, felt odd sensations of fingers pulling his hair and hands brushing his cheeks. These strange phenomena continued throughout other sessions: Roger experienced sensations of cold, heard thumps, and witnessed the movement of objects.

Roger must have had some degree of mediumistic ability all along, which perhaps awakened within him as a result of attending the séances, because he soon began to produce automatic writing. While outside the circle, moreover, he began to experience the same odd sensations of someone touching his hair and face. He was soon diagnosed with schizophrenia. The treatment he received from a Jungian psychiatrist proved beneficial, though it did have one drawback – as his psychotic symptoms started to recede, there began, around him, typical poltergeist activity, which followed him wherever he went. Doors would fly open in his presence, raps would sound, and he was constantly touched. On a number of occasions, his head was also grasped and turned.

Seeking further help, Roger became acquainted with Mary Williams. During their first session together, Roger and Williams both heard loud and random poltergeist raps. Mysterious raps were heard during later sessions as well. At one point, says Williams, while Roger was relating a dream, "the cupboard door in front of us opened slowly and silently." When, on one occasion, he felt the poltergeist trying to turn his head, Williams actually saw "his neck muscles straining, as if resisting a powerful force."

Williams explains: "Meanwhile the poltergeist was playing up every time he went to see his girlfriend, and tormented her in his absence. It tormented him too at night. It would get hold of him in bed, and hold him fast while it tickled his face and tugged his hair. And his mother was hearing raps daily...After a few weeks he reported that the last time the poltergeist had got hold of him, it had seemed more gentle and had actually moved him into a more comfortable position. He did not resist this time, and let it hold him...It was only a few days later that it materialized again, and it was its last appearance. It came to him in bed and lay beside him. He felt it pressing up against his side, then it seemed to be merging with him, and he experienced it as loving and gave himself to it."

Williams's take on the case is that Roger was essentially denying part of himself. He was, she points out, highly promiscuous, yet unable to achieve full sexual satisfaction in his relationships. After giving himself to the entity, or "merging" with the entity, however, his sex life became a happy one, and he was able to experience full orgasm. No longer was he bothered by poltergeist activity; nor did the "succubus" return. Gooch uses the case as an example of "what can be achieved by the human subjective mind manipulating and actualizing itself in the external, objective universe around it," as well as evidence that there is a link between poltergeist activity and succubi/incubi encounters.

If you are irresponsible enough to participate in séances and the like – so as to contact your relatives on "the other side," or because you desire entertainment – perhaps you deserve what you get. But attempting to develop mediumistic powers is even worse and is really asking for trouble. During the heyday of spiritualism (not to be confused with Kardec's Spiritism), dabbling in automatic writing and other forms of mediumship was quite common, and many a bored housewife became mentally ill as a result. Specific cases of this, of people having their sanity threatened by troublesome discarnate entities, can be found in *The Infinite Bound-*

ary: Spirit Possession, Madness, and Multiple Personality, written by the late, great parapsychologist D. Scott Rogo, whose mysterious death (he was found stabbed to death in his Los Angeles home in 1990, aged 40) is further proof that those who dedicate their lives to paranormal research often meet a tragic fate.

There can be no doubt whatsoever that the SP phenomenon has a "spiritual" side, and that this may be its predominant aspect. It also has a physiological side, which we have already touched upon, but which doesn't overly concern us in this study. The SP phenomenon has its roots in the astral realm, the invisible realm, and so, should we wish to get to the heart of the matter, we need to explore it at that level.

In our quest to better understand the SP phenomenon, as well its various "offshoots," such as OBEs, LDs, poltergeist hauntings, etc., the occult/shamanic perspective has served us well – and will continue to do so. Both the occultist and the shaman have an answer to the cause of SP attacks. They know that discarnate entities are partly to blame. They realize, moreover, that perception is dependent on one's state of consciousness, and that, more specifically, the hypnagogic and hypnopompic states are doorways into the "spirit realm." For them, reality is not limited to what we can perceive with our five senses but stretches further outward to that which lies "beyond the veil."

In many indigenous cultures throughout the world, in which shamanistic beliefs and practices play an important role, it's widely believed that during sleep the soul leaves the body and goes wandering, and, further, that in this state the person is particularly vulnerable to the influence of spirits. In a compelling paper titled "Eskimo Sleep Paralysis," the authors, Joseph D. Bloom and Richard D. Gelardin, explain how the Eskimo people of Alaska perceive the SP phenomenon. According to a thirty-year-old Eskimo woman who first experienced SP as a child and was clearly a chronic SP sufferer, the phenomenon, her grandparents had told her, was caused by "a soul trying to take possession of me." They urged her to "fight" the experiences.

Bloom and Gelardin discovered that SP is well known among the Eskimo and is discussed openly; just about everyone has heard of the phenomenon and many have experienced it first-hand. The Eskimo believe, explain the authors, "that when people are entering sleep, sleeping, or emerging from sleep, they are more susceptible to influences from the spirit world...One of the informants felt that if an individual did not believe in the spirit world he would be challenged; 'a spirit would come to you and make you realize that there are spirits.'" This strikes me as a comment worthy of discussion, for it seems to me that some of the spirits who make their presence known during SP attacks are simply trying to let you know that they exist, and that the "spirit realm" is real.

The authors were told that the paralysis one experiences is caused by the soul leaving the body, and that, if this condition persists, death can result. (We know this to be false, of course, as bodily paralysis is a natural part of the REM state.) According to another explanation the authors were given, paralysis occurs because a spirit has temporarily possessed the person; the spirit has entered their body and is controlling it. In my view, these explanations, although ostensibly silly and superstitious, are far more logical and make much more sense than the official "enlightened" explanation that we are all expected to agree with – that SP attacks are meaningless "neurological glitches" and should not be given much thought.

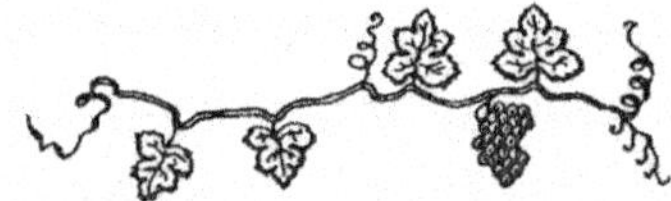

One of the greatest experts on "psychic attacks" was the advanced British occultist Dion Fortune. Born Violet Mary Firth (1890-1946) in Bryn-y-Bia, Llandudno, Wales, Fortune reported visions of Atlantis at age four and is said to have developed mediumistic abilities in her twentieth year. After attending courses in psychology and psychotherapy at the University of London, she practiced for some time as a lay psychotherapist. Drawn to the occult, she joined the Theosophical Society and was later initiated into the London Temple of The Alpha et Omega (formerly named The Hermetic Order of the Golden Dawn). Fortune eventually founded her own magical order, The Society of the Inner Light. Her works include a number of novels and short stories, but she is best remembered for her non-fiction books on magical subjects, such as *The Cosmic Doctrine*, *The Mystical Qabalah*, and the aforementioned *Psychic Self-Defence*, all of them classics in their field.

Like many great occultists, Fortune is supposed to have had access to the "Akashic Records," that great storehouse of knowledge encoded in the aether. She supposedly drew from this knowledge, channeling it into her literary work. Thus many of her books almost "wrote themselves." An occultist of the highest order who like Rudolf Steiner was firmly of the right-hand path, not the left, Fortune is credited with contributing to the revival of the Mystery Tradition of the West and is recognized as one of the most significant figures of 20th century esoteric thought.

Fortune was well aware that occult powers can be used to achieve harmful ends, as well as good. Knowledge in the wrong hands, occult or otherwise, can be a very dangerous thing. For an occult attack to be possible, for there to be an "entrance to the soul," the aura of the victim has to be pierced, says Fortune, and this always occurs from within, "by the response of fear or desire going out towards the attacking entity." One is immediately reminded of the Enfield poltergeist case and the damaged and leaking auras of Janet and her mother.

In the event of a psychic attack, it's important, says Fortune, to keep your cool and not let your emotions get the better of yourself in order to ensure that your aura remains strong, healthy, and impenetrable. It's a well-known fact that those who suffer from anxiety and depression often feel tired and lethargic, while those who remain optimistic and happy have an abundance of energy. Colin Wilson once said, "We go around leaking energy in the same way that someone who has slashed their wrists would go around leaking blood."

According to Fortune, it's possible for a trained occultist to project their etheric body, or etheric double, at will, and to use it as a "weapon" of "psychic attack." These attacks are usually carried out at night, she says, while the victim is asleep and therefore psychically vulnerable. "If there is a definite psychic attack of sufficient force to make itself noticeable at all," she writes, "there soon begin to appear characteristic dreams. These may include a sense of weight upon the chest, as if someone were kneeling on the sleeper." This effect, she says, far from being hallucinatory, is actually caused by a concentration of etheric substance or ectoplasm; she defines an etheric substance as an intermediary substance between mind and matter. "Occultists maintain that mind affects body by means of the etheric double," she explains. The etheric body is similar in nature to, though not the same as, the perispirit of the Spiritists.

Fortune defines ectoplasm as an intermediary substance between the etheric body and the physical body, calling it "the raw material out of which dense matter is condensed." Apparently, a medium can project this substance in the form of either "long rods" or "nebulous clouds," which they can then use to affect matter directly, or to create materializations of various kinds.

Throughout *Psychic Self-Defence*, Fortune mentions *two* subtle bodies – the etheric and the astral – but doesn't sufficiently explain the differences between them, resulting in much confusion. Sometimes occultists use these terms interchangeably, indicating that they refer to exactly the same thing, but this is not true. According to occult thought, the aura is said to comprise a number of subtle bodies, the least subtle of which is the etheric body. The etheric body is a double or blueprint of the physical body, duplicating it in all its parts and organs. It surrounds and interpenetrates the physical body, and, as Constable demonstrates in *The Cosmic Pulse of Life*, "it is perceivable by any person of normal vision who uses the correct techniques."

Next up from the etheric body, and of an even more subtle constitution, is the astral body, which is said to be the seat of consciousness and of the emotions. The astral body is known by the Spiritists as the perispirit. Plants, animals, and humans all possess etheric bodies, but only animals and humans possess astral bodies. "The astral body is of emotional substance," explains Constable, "and not accessible to physical detection like the etheric body and its radiation." It has been said that only those with some degree of psychic ability can perceive this vehicle.

In *Psychic Self-Defence*, Fortune mentions the time she was subjected to a series of psychic attacks by a woman she calls Miss L., whom she describes as neurotic, "morbidly humanitarian," and fastidious, yet outwardly kind and normal. Fortune had just taken up residence at an occult college "in the sandy fastnesses of the Hampshire barrens," and, knowing Miss L. was keen to get away from the city, asked if she might like to stay at the college too, and help out with the domestic duties there. Miss L. took up the offer, arriving at the college several days after Fortune.

That same night, Fortune was awakened by a "nightmare" and "struggled with a weight on my chest." Her bedroom, she says, "seemed full of evil." However, she managed to purify the atmosphere in the room by performing a simple banishing ritual. The next morning, while breakfasting with the other members of the community, she was surprised to learn that she wasn't the only one whose night had been disturbed – five or six others had also experienced "nightmares." While Fortune and the others were comparing experiences, Mrs. L. became angry, telling them not to talk about such "unwholesome" things. For the next few days, the "nightmares" continued, afflicting various members of the community. These experiences, they agreed, were probably brought about by indigestion, "caused by the village baker's version of war bread."

The next day, Fortune and Miss L. had an argument after Miss L. confessed to Fortune that she had a "crush" on her. Being the hard-headed woman that she was and having "a constitutional repulsion for crushes," it's little wonder that Fortune responded in such a way as to upset Miss L. (One can gather from her writing that Fortune was a strong and practical woman who had little time for other people's nonsense. As for her use of the word "crush," one can only assume that it was used to denote a feeling of romantic attraction.) That night, Fortune experienced "one of the most violent nightmares I have had in my life, waking from sleep with a terrible sense of oppression on my chest, as if someone were holding me down or lying upon me." What she describes next is bound to bring a smile to the reader's face: "I saw distinctly the head of Miss L., reduced to the size of an orange, floating in the air at the foot of my bed, and snapping its teeth at me. It was the most malignant thing I have ever seen."

Not long afterwards, while working peacefully in the kitchen together, a sudden change came over Miss L., and she became, in Fortune's words, "as mad as a March hare." In what sounds like something conceived by the warped minds of Rik Mayall and Adrian Edmondson (writers and stars of the British slapstick sitcom *Bottom*), Miss L. picked up a large carving knife and began chasing Fortune around the kitchen. Luckily, writes Fortune, "I had in my hands a large saucepan full of freshly boiled greens, and I used this as a weapon of defense..." Given the fact that Miss L. actually slashed at her with the knife, it's lucky that Fortune wasn't injured. Right in the middle of the incident, the head of the community entered the room, and Miss L. suddenly ceased what she was doing.

The head of the community, whom Fortune refers to as "Z," (and who many believe was probably John William Brodie-Innes, a leading member of the Golden Dawn's temple in Edinburgh), was able to read the situation and knew how best to handle Miss L. Every night he "sealed the threshold" of Miss L's room with the pentagram so that nothing could get out. He also sealed his own room, so that nothing could get in. For those unfamiliar with the occult significance of the five-pointed star, it is, simply put, a symbol of protection and purification, provided of course that it's positioned correctly with one point facing up. An inverted pentagram, which has two points facing up, signifies chaos and evil. According to the famous French occultist Eliphas Levi, the pentagram "exercises a great influence upon spirits and terrifies phantoms."

The rituals performed by Z appeared to have a positive effect on Miss L. Over the course of a few weeks, her moods stabilized, and no more incidents of psychic attack were reported. She confessed to everyone that she had memories of dealings with black magic in previous lives and, as a child, would often daydream that she was a witch, able to use her powers to get revenge on those who had wronged her – even willing their deaths. Sometimes, she said, she would visualize herself standing before people she was angry with, projecting negative energy towards them. But this, she added, was not entirely her fault, for she felt as though she were two separate people – one compassionate and spiritual, the other cruel, petty, and sadistic. Whenever she became cross, upset, or exhausted, the latter "personality" would rise to the surface and in a sense take over. She would then indulge in acts of psychic attack, hence the "nightmares" experienced by Fortune and the other members of the community.

According to Fortune, not only is it possible to use your etheric body as a weapon of psychic attack, it's also possible to create, from your etheric body, a kind of "artificial ghost." Those who have read Alexandra David-Neel's *Magic and Mystery in Tibet* (1929) will be familiar with the concept of tulpas, or "thought-forms." These etheric beings, created through intense visualization, are able to take on a life of their own and may cause problems for the individual (or individuals) who created them. David-Neel claims to have been "haunted" by a tulpa she brought into being – a jolly monk – which she ended up having to destroy.

In *Psychic Self-Defence*, Fortune distinguishes between "thought-forms" and what she calls "artificial elementals," explaining that the latter, unlike the former, "possess a distinct and independent life of their own..." In accordance with Fortune's terminology, then, David-Neel's monk was really an artificial elemental. "The life of these creatures is akin to that of an electric battery," she explains, "it slowly leaks out by means of radiation, and unless recharged periodically, will finally weaken and die out." It almost sounds as though Fortune is writing about the poltergeist, which could also be compared to a type of rechargeable battery (but one with a limited lifespan, because poltergeists always lose their power eventually). Provided such beings exist, it would not be unreasonable to suppose that some poltergeist disturbances are caused by artificial elementals.

It sometimes happens, says Fortune, that these beings are created unintentionally. As an example, she describes an unpleasant experience of her own, which occurred at a time when she was angry with someone who had wronged her. While lying in bed one afternoon, "brooding over my resentment," she "drifted towards the borders of sleep," and began thinking of the Norse wolf-monster Fenrir. "Immediately I felt a curious drawing-out sensation from my solar plexus, and there materialized beside me on the bed a large wolf." She describes its "ectoplasmic form" as grey and colorless.

She mentions, moreover, that it possessed weight, and that she could feel its back pressing against her body. At the time the "materialization" took place, Fortune was obviously in the hypnagogic state – a state in which "the etheric double readily extrudes."

Knowing that the creature was essentially under her control, "provided I did not panic" and that "it was really a part of myself extruded," Fortune attempted to get the upper hand on the beast by treating it like a naughty pet. She pushed it off the bed with her elbow, saying "If you can't behave yourself, you will just have to go on the floor." The creature then changed from a wolf into a dog, and she saw it exit through a section of the wall that had faded away. The following morning, a woman who lived in the same house said her sleep had been disturbed by dreams of wolves, and that she had awoken to see the shining eyes of a wild animal.

Before the situation got out of control and the creature was able to "sever the psychic navel cord that connected it to my solar plexus," Fortune managed to summon the creature and absorb it back into herself, which involved drawing the life out of it, "as if sucking lemonade up a straw." This process, she says, was a most unpleasant and taxing one because she had to take on all the negative emotions that had gone into constructing the creature. "I felt the most furious impulses to go berserk..." By the end of it, she was bathed in perspiration.

According to Fortune, the role that thought-forms play in psychic disturbances should not be overlooked. It's possible, she says, for a person to be "haunted" by their own thought-forms, because, whatever "we extrude from our auras, unless absorbed by the object to which they are directed, will return to us in due course." As an extreme example of this, she mentions how schizophrenics (although she does not refer to them as such) think themselves to be persecuted by invisible beings, when, in actual fact, although these "beings" have a partially objective existence, they are actually thought-forms exuded from the aura of the patient. They are, in other words, the dissociated complex of the patient that has taken on a life of its own. "A psychic who investigates such a case can very often see the alleged entities just where the lunatic says they are." Destroying these entities, she says, does not cure the patient but only offers them temporary relief – temporary because "unless the cause of the illness can be dealt with, a fresh batch of thought-forms is built up as soon as the original ones are destroyed."

Like many great spiritual teachers, Fortune was of the opinion that our thoughts are far more powerful than we assume, and that negative thoughts, when sufficiently concentrated, can act as a kind of "psychic poison." It could be said that we all live inside our own minds, which for many people is a very confined, air-tight "space," much like a pantry. According to this analogy (and I apologize to the reader if it sounds a little rude), the seriously mentally ill, particularly the hallucinating schizophrenic, could be likened to a man with very bad flatulence, trapped inside a pantry, each negative thought being a particularly offensive fart. The more the man farts, the more he begins to notice the stink. To some extent, we all "choke" on our own negative energies.

In *Psychic Self-Defence*, Fortune stresses that people must take responsibility for their own thoughts, conscious or unconscious, instead of placing the blame of "psychic attack" on something or someone else. Indeed, perhaps many SP experiences can be explained as a result of negative thought-forms that have, in Fortune's words, "returned home to roost."

It's natural for the sexually repressed and the sexually starved, such as teenage boys who are undergoing puberty, to spend much time thinking about sex, which may involve playing out certain fantasies in their mind. A young man, for instance, may be so obsessed with a woman whom he wishes to bed that he'll spend all night thinking about her, imagining the seduction, in great detail, in his mind. As he indulges in these masturbatory fantasies, working himself into a state of sexual fever, he might, perhaps, drift into the hypnagogic state.

If it's true what Fortune says about the period between sleeping and waking being a condition "in which the etheric double readily extrudes," then it's quite possible that the young man's sexual fantasies will "come alive," becoming thought-forms, and that these thought-forms will eventually return to "haunt" him. Perhaps, in certain cases, in order to sustain their existence, these thought-forms act like energy vampires, attacking the young man in his sleep and sucking away his vitality. Maybe some cases of incubi and succubi attacks can be explained in this way.

Psychic Self-Defence includes a chapter on vampirism. However, the types of vampires Fortune describes are not blood-drinking humans, but rather, earth-bound souls who have avoided the "second death" – in other words, the disintegration of the astral body – and have "maintained themselves in the etheric double" by vampirizing the living. Apparently, those who have been attacked by such beings having been depleted of vital energy to a life-threatening degree, become energy vampires themselves, stealing from others the energy they need. It sometimes happens, says Fortune, that the entity attaches itself permanently to its human vampire victim, much like a parasite, stealing the energy from its victim that he himself has stolen from other people.

Keeping in mind that *Psychic Self-Defence* was first published in the 1930s, and that Fortune herself, although spiritually wise, was perhaps a little superstitious, she explains that those with vampiric tendencies "develop abnormally long and sharp canine teeth." This could very well be true, but I think it highly unlikely. I myself have long, sharp canine teeth, and many people have commented that they resemble those of a typical movie vampire. I can assure the reader, however, that the only vital energy I consume is my own! Were I a vampire, it would mean that the English pop star David Bowie is also a vampire – or maybe a vampire no more, seeing as he recently lost those prominent canine teeth.

While Miss L. was staying at the college, many of the residents were afflicted by "exceedingly bad 'mosquito bites.'" Fortune explains: "The bites themselves were not poisonous, but the stabs were of such a nature that they bled freely. I remember waking up one morning to find a patch of blood the size of the palm of my hand on the pillow." Following a disturbed sleep, I too have noticed the presence of such marks on my pillow and bedclothes, but of a size far smaller than that of a palm. Normal mosquito bites could not possibly have caused them. Interestingly, reports of mysterious bloodstains also appear in cases of alien abduction, as do chronic nosebleeds, abductees claiming that they have them fairly often.

According to occult thought, blood, being a vital fluid, contains a large amount of ectoplasm or etheric substance. When shed, "this ectoplasm readily separates from the congealing blood and thus becomes available for materializations," explains Fortune in her book *Sane Occultism*. However, she adds, only beings of a very low class make use of blood in this way, such as some of the fearsome deities who are worshipped by primitive peoples, whereby an animal will be slaughtered and offered as a sacrifice. "Any strong emotion is a source of astral energy, and fear and pain are no exceptions to the rule," she adds. That fear is a source of "food" for lower astral entities makes perfect sense in light of how the SP victim feels during a typical attack. These experiences, more than anything else, scare people out of their absolute wits. Could it be that the entities behind SP attacks are trying to induce fear in their victims so as to feast on their "astral energy"? Bear in mind, too, that stress and anxiety are known to contribute towards SP attacks.

In certain Tibetan Buddhist ceremonies, offerings are made to the beings that inhabit the hungry ghost realm. Usually these offerings are of food and drink, although particular types of smoke are also used. At the Buddhist center where I used to live, the Buddhists would sometimes build a fire inside an old bathtub, placing bundles of fresh pine needles on top of the hot coals. As the ceremony was being performed, the scented smoke from these smoldering pine needles would waft around the center, providing nourishment, I suppose, for swarms of hungry ghosts who had gathered in the vicinity. In western ceremonial magic, incense and other volatile substances are sometimes burnt as a means of allowing entities to manifest – in this case, entities slightly more evolved than the kind that have a penchant for blood. When burnt, says Fortune, these substances release "ethers" – and this is what the entities make use of.

To be honest, I have often questioned the judiciousness and safety of Tibetan Buddhist hungry ghost offerings. Assuming that spirits are in fact drawn to offerings of food, smoke, and other substances, does it really seem wise to attract these astral degenerates? Would such actions not place you at risk of psychic attack, particularly the SP sufferer, who, psychically speaking, is of a much more sensitive constitution than the average man? This is not to say, of course, that I don't believe in practicing compassion; I'm all for it, and when it comes to troubled earthbound spirits, my heart overflows with compassion. I have compassion for wild animals too, but if I happened to encounter a hungry lion while walking in the savannah, I wouldn't invite it back to my house for supper. I'd leave it well alone. And if it didn't leave me alone, I'd run like a man possessed (pun intended)!

To prove I'm not picking on the Buddhists, I should explain that I consider all dealings with spirits potentially dangerous. It makes little difference if these dealings take the form of mediumistic sessions, Ouija board experiments, or hungry ghost offerings – the risk of attracting unwholesome entities is too great. To give the Tibetan Buddhists their due, I should say that they, in comparison to those of the western esoteric tradition, do not interact with spirits very much at all and generally believe it best to refrain from such practices as mediumship, for example.

In *Psychic Self-Defence*, Fortune discusses the various types of physical manifestations that can occur during a psychic attack. Some of the phenomena she lists are as follows: lights, "usually taking the form of dim balls of luminous mist, drifting like soap bubbles"; distinctive odors; the movement of light objects, which are sometimes thrown about the room; and inexplicable noises, "usually creakings, thuds, or more rarely bell-like notes or wailing sounds." Fortune adds: "If actual words are heard, auditory hallucinations should be suspected, for in the absence of a medium, spirit messages are given to the inner ear, not to the auditory nerve."

These details are of great significance to this study because they confirm everything we've learned so far about poltergeist disturbances. Seeing as Fortune states that a medium needs to be present for "spirit messages" to be heard by normal means, this would seem to suggest that, like the Spiritists, she was aware of the fact that the focus of a poltergeist disturbance is an unconscious medium. Perhaps she was familiar with *The Mediums' Book*. Or maybe she came to this conclusion on her own. Whatever the case, it's now time we took a closer look at the phenomenon of "spirit messages" or auditory hallucinations.

CHAPTER 12

Those Troublesome Voices

One day, the Thing [the poltergeist] even gave Mrs. Harper [Peggy Hodgson] a helping hand, for a change, with her cooking. She was making a cake, and just about to pour the sugar into the mixing bowl, when she distinctly heard a voice in her ear saying: 'You haven't got enough sugar there, Mum!' It sounded like one of the Voices, but all the children were out of the house. And sure enough, when she checked, she found she had indeed not got enough sugar for her usual recipe. – Guy Lyon Playfair, *This House is Haunted: The Investigation into the Enfield Poltergeist*

There are, it seems, two main ways that spirits can manifest. I describe these two ways as "internally" and "externally." The terms subjectively and objectively would also suffice. The poltergeist activity that surrounded Roger – as described in the previous chapter – is a good example of an external manifestation, while Roger's "succubi" encounter is a good example of an internal manifestation. Clearly, most SP attacks occur on an internal level.

It would be logical to assume that cases of spirit possession start with internal manifestations, and, as the spirit gains a firmer grip on its victim's mind, external manifestations then develop. This, however, is not always the case. Spirits who, in Fortune's words, "have gained a foothold on the physical plane" are not necessarily more powerful or dangerous than spirits who are confined to their own realm. In Roger's case, the spirit that bothered him first manifested as a poltergeist, then later as a "succubus" – not the other way around.

The reader will have noticed that the types of phenomena experienced by SP sufferers – these of course being internal manifestations – have much in common with the types of phenomena that occur when the "spirit world breaks through" and, for example, poltergeist disturbances erupt. In other words, internal manifestations have much in common with external manifestations. In both cases, many of the same types of sounds are heard: footsteps, raps, slamming doors, and one's name being called, for example. While in the hypnagogic state, for instance, Martyn would often hear "knocks, sometimes regularly spaced, one – two – three, and also less determinate thumps." These rapping/knocking sounds are so common to poltergeist disturbances as to be a trademark of the phenomenon. In the Enfield case, loud and persistent knocking sounds were heard frequently.

Similarities between internal manifestations and external manifestations are not limited to sound. In both cases, many of the same types of sensations are felt. For example, some SP sufferers, myself included, report the sensation of having their bed shaken or rocked back and forth. And as we know, poltergeists enjoy shaking and moving beds around, particularly the one belonging to the agent. During a violent SP attack, it's not uncommon to be choked by an evil spirit, a phenomenon also reported by poltergeist victims.

There is one internal manifestation that deserves further exploration – auditory hallucinations. Recall what Fortune said regarding physical manifestations in psychic attacks: "If actual words are heard, auditory hallucinations should be suspected, for in the absence of a medium, spirit messages are given to the inner ear, not to the auditory nerve." The inner ear is the innermost part of the ear from which sound waves are transmitted to the brain as nerve impulses. Connecting the inner ear with the brain is the auditory nerve, which has two branches, one of which carries the sensation of sound to the brain, while the other is involved in maintaining balance. However, Fortune is referring, not to a part of the physical ear, but to a spiritual faculty of sorts. To hear with your inner ear is to "hear" psychically or spiritually.

There are, according to *The Mediums' Book*, "two very distinct ways in which spirit-sounds are perceived; they are sometimes heard by a sort of interior hearing, in which case, although the words heard are clear and distinct, they are not of a physical nature; at other times, these voices are perceived as something exterior to ourselves, and appear to be as distinctly articulated as though spoken by a person at our side."

Now it would appear that these two ways of perceiving "spirit sounds" both involve the use of one's "inner ear," though perhaps this applies more to the former – "a sort of interior hearing" – than to the latter. SP sufferers experience auditory hallucinations in both an interior fashion and an exterior fashion, though mainly the latter. That *The Mediums' Book* accurately identifies these two different types of voices is beyond remarkable; it offers further evidence in support of the spirit hypothesis put forward here.

Speaking of auditory hallucinations, I experienced a new type this morning, before getting up to write the current chapter. I woke up rather late, and was lying in bed, relaxing. Feeling lazy, I was unable to force myself out of bed. After a while, I drifted into a state of deep and pleasant relaxation. I then heard a voice in my head, which interrupted my train of thought. It told me to "Go to sleep." The voice was male and sounded distinctly Australian. Had I, perhaps, entered the hypnagogic state? Most likely. Never before have I experienced an auditory hallucination while feeling so awake.

The voice seemed thought-like, was not particularly loud, and unlike most of those I've heard, did not emanate from outside my head. One could describe it as a "foreign thought," in the sense that it clearly did not belong to the other thoughts I was having, nor did it seem to originate from my own mind. *The Spirits' Book* discusses this matter – about how (usually when our senses have "grown torpid") we sometimes "seem to hear within ourselves words distinctly pronounced, but having no connection with what we are thinking of." When this occurs, the book explains, it occasionally means that we've managed to pick up, "the faint echo of the utterance of a spirit who wishes to communicate with you."

Most of us assume that the mentally ill, particularly the psychotic, are the only ones who hear voices, but this is simply not true. Even people with good mental health will sometimes report such experiences. In a study conducted in 1889 by the Society for Psychical Research (SPR), involving 17,000 interviewees from England, Russia, and Brazil, all of them "normal" adults, the following question was asked: "Have you ever, when believing yourself to be completely awake, had a vivid impression of seeing or being touched by a living being or inanimate object, or of hearing a voice: which impression, so far as you could discover, was not due to any external cause?" Nearly 10 percent of the respondents answered yes, and of those 2.9 percent said their hallucination took the form of a phantom voice.

More than a hundred years later, Professor Allen Y. Tien carried out a similar survey involving 15,000 people from Baltimore, St. Louis, and Los Angeles. Tien discovered that voices are heard regularly by 2.3 percent of the general population. Other contemporary studies on the prevalence of auditory hallucinations within the general population have yielded similar results. Of course, those most likely to hear voices are people who suffer from some kind of psychosis. According to Ralph Hoffman, a professor of psychiatry at Yale University, the condition affects 70 percent of patients with schizophrenia and 15 percent of patients with mood disorders. Non-psychotic conditions and diagnoses, such as depression and post-traumatic stress disorder, can also bring about auditory hallucinations.

In his celebrated 1976 work *The Origin of Consciousness in the Break-*

down of the Bicameral Mind, the late Julian Jaynes, a Princeton University psychologist, put forward the remarkable theory that ancient man possessed a different state of consciousness to that of modern man and was much like a modern-day schizophrenic who hears voices ordering him what to do. These auditory hallucinations, he says, were commonly thought to be the voice of God, or the gods, but were actually produced by the right hemisphere of the brain – which in ancient man was less connected to its other half, the left brain, than it is today. ("Bicameral" means having two compartments.) If this theory is correct, it might help explain why characters in the *Old Testament* and the *Iliad* are always being counseled by "divine voices," and why in both of these texts and others written during the same period no mention is made of any kind of cognitive processes, such as introspection.

The left brain and the right brain are basically two different "personalities," the left being likened to a scientist and the right an artist. The left hemisphere, which is the more dominant of the two, is logical, analytical, and verbal, while the right is creative, holistic, and nonverbal. Joining the two hemispheres is a bridge of nerve fibers called the corpus callosum; without it, they would not be able to communicate with each other. Studies have shown that musicians have significantly larger corpora callosa than non-musicians. It also tends to be slightly larger in left-handed people than right-handed people. Some have speculated, mainly fringe writers, that the right hemisphere is the home of the unconscious mind. But, pleasing and logical though this theory sounds, very little evidence exists to support it.

In some extreme cases, to reduce the severity of seizures experienced by epileptic patients, an operation is performed whereby the corpus callosum is severed. This is called a corpus callosum section, or corpus callosotomy. Afterwards, a most peculiar thing occurs. The two hemispheres of the brain – the left hemisphere (which controls the right side of the body) and the right hemisphere (which controls the left side of the body) – start to have "disagreements" over certain issues as the patient becomes, in a sense, two separate people. With some split-brain patients, their left hemisphere will express one opinion, and their right hemisphere will express the complete opposite. One patient who was angry at his wife tried to strike her with his left hand, while his right hand, in an attempt to protect her, held it back.

Experiments have been performed in which split-brain patients were shown pictures of nudes. When only their right hemispheres viewed the images (their left eyes), the patients were found to grin or blush in embarrassment. When asked to explain their reactions, the patients were unable to do so. Experiments such as this have been used as evidence to support the "right hemisphere unconscious mind theory" (if one could call it such). It should be noted, however, that when the pictures were shown to the patients' left hemispheres (their right eyes), they also blushed or grinned and, unlike before, were able to explain why. So, even though the right cerebral hemisphere is nonverbal, it would be incorrect to regard it as "unconscious." The cerebrum, which comprises both hemispheres, is considered to be the seat of conscious mental processes – namely, the physical location of the conscious, cognitive mind.

If, argues Gooch in *The Origins of Psychic Phenomena*, the right cerebral hemisphere is the home of the unconscious mind, a sleeping person should exhibit electrical activity exclusively, or primarily, in this region of the brain. Furthermore, the same results should be present in someone who was meditating – another activity related to the unconscious mind. In both instances, however, there is an equal amount of, and the same kind of, electrical activity in both regions of the brain. Gooch proposes that the cerebellum – or "little brain" – is the physical seat of the unconscious mind. He points out that strong evidence exists to suggest that the cerebellum is directly responsible for the function of dreaming. Women, he says, who are generally more psychic than men, have larger cerebella, as confirmed by brain imaging techniques.

As evidence of the fact that perfectly healthy people, though generally under conditions of stress, can sometimes hear disembodied voices, Jaynes describes an experience of his own. It happened in his late twenties, while living alone in Boston. He had been studying for about a week, pondering the question "of what knowledge is and how we can know anything at all," when, one afternoon, in a state of "intellectual despair," he lay down on the couch (and presumably drifted into a hypnagogic state). He heard "a firm, distinct loud voice from my upper right which said, 'Include the knower in the known!' The voice had had an exact location. No one was there! Not even behind the wall where I sheepishly looked."

One perfectly sane young woman, the wife of a biologist, told Jaynes she had regular conversations with her dead mother while making the beds in the morning. But, unlike the type of conversations that a schizophrenic might have with one of their "voices," these were "long, informative, and pleasant." When the woman's husband found out about this, he was rather shocked, to say the least. Hearing voices is, after all, thought to be something that only the mentally ill experience, not perfectly functioning members of society. Those who have these experiences, in some cases regularly since early-adolescence, learn to keep their mouths shut – and with good reason, too, for who would like to be diagnosed with schizophrenia.

In his remarkable book about the history, science, and meaning of auditory hallucinations, *Muses, Madmen, and Prophets*, American journalist Daniel B. Smith relates how his father, Leonard, and his grandfather both heard voices for most of their lives but managed to hide their condition for many years from everyone they knew, including their relatives. In 1995, when Daniel was seventeen years old, he and his brother helped edit and type up a manuscript that their grandfather had written – a memoir entitled *The Smith Family Chronicles*. It took, in total, a week of afternoons.

When the task was done, they printed off a copy and handed it to Leonard. For reasons not known at the time, one section of the book sent their normally unemotional father into a rage. "He railed at a great injustice that had been done to him. He fumed and festered over time wasted and anguish unnecessarily endured." He eventually flew to Florida to confront Daniel's grandfather.

The section in the memoir that sparked his father's rage was titled "Voices." Part of it reads: "I have always heard them, but it took some time for me to recognize that they had a significance. Mostly they appeared when there was a decision-making problem…When, after a decision was made, incorrectly, I would think back in retrospect and recall that a voice in my head told me the proper thing to do…Mother and I have a regular gin game with friends from the mountains…When it is my turn to discard a card from my hand, invariably, an inner voice will tell me that he needs the card. I have proven this, time and time again, by holding back the voice card discarded, but later throwing it, he always picks up and needs this card."

The reason Leonard reacted the way he did was that he too had heard voices – since the age of thirteen, in fact – yet was told nothing of his father's experiences. For twenty-five years, Leonard told no one about the voices he heard on a regular basis, most of which issued simple commands, telling him, for instance, "to move a glass from one side of the table to the other or to use a specific token in a specific subway turnstile." He considered the voices extremely undesirable, though they were neither cruel nor harsh, and wanted nothing more than to be rid of them.

At one point in Leonard's life, they became unbearable, and he suffered a nervous breakdown. It was then that he told his wife about them.

He admitted himself to the psychiatric ward of a nearby hospital and returned home a couple of weeks later. In his absence, the law firm he worked for had dismissed him, branding him mentally unfit, while the family he loved "was on the brink of dissolution." Fortunately, explains Smith, his father's mental health improved, and he soon got his life back together again. "But," he adds, "the *Chronicles* made him feel that his long struggle might have been avoided... My father felt that he had been denied his salvation."

That Leonard and his father had both heard voices seems to suggest that there was a genetic component to their condition – whatever their condition may have been exactly. But to say that they both had the same condition would be inaccurate. In Leonard's case, the voices were an unwanted nuisance, and, in Daniel's words, "caused him profound distress." And in his father's case, the voices were subtle and helpful and could even be described as a kind of intuition. Explaining this disparity is no easy task. Leonard was apparently diagnosed with "major depression with psychotic features." He certainly did not suffer from schizophrenia; neither did his father. What, then, was the cause of their voices? Had their minds been invaded by spirits?

Referring to the voices heard by schizophrenic patients, Jaynes writes: "They converse, threaten, curse, criticize, consult, often in short sentences. They admonish, console, mock, command, or sometimes simply announce everything that's happening. They yell, whine, sneer, and vary from the slightest whisper to a thunderous shout. Often the voices take on some special peculiarity, such as speaking very slowly, scanning, rhyming, or in rhymes, or even in foreign languages. There may be one particular voice, more often a few voices, and occasionally many." Colin Wilson, in his book *Afterlife,* observes: "There is no reason, of course, why 'phantom voices' should not sound like those of a normal person. But it seems to be a fact that most of them don't."

"When the illness is most severe," continues Jaynes, "the voices are loudest and come from outside; when least severe, voices often tend to be internal whispers..." This brings us back to the "two very distinct ways in which spirit-sounds are perceived," as explained in *The Mediums' Book* – one "a sort of interior hearing," the other "exterior to ourselves...as though spoken by a person at our side." As we know, SP sufferers also hear voices in both of these manners. That the voices of schizophrenics vary in volume and intensity depending on the severity of the illness at the time lends support to my "tuning theory," mentioned in a previous chapter. Using the analogy of a radio picking up a station, I explained that when a spirit wishes to communicate with a person, the process is one of correct tuning.

Clearly, the auditory hallucinations of SP sufferers and schizophrenics are not that dissimilar. Further evidence of this can be found in a fascinating paper by J. Allan Cheyne, entitled "The Ominous Numinous: Sensed Presence and Other Hallucinations." In it he explains that the voices of SP sufferers are "often described as 'gibberish,' 'garbled,' or 'foreign sounding.' In cases in which the voices are comprehensible their messages are typically simple and direct. The voices may simply call out the sleeper's name, but more often, they utter a threat, warning, command or a cry for help."

I've previously cited numerous descriptions of these voices written by SP sufferers. Cheyne's paper mentions several more examples:

- "When I awoke to the women's voice telling me I was going to die if I didn't wake up."
- "The first time, when I was on my side, I heard heavy breathing. The second time, when I was lying on my back, I heard an evil voice saying, "I'm going to get you now; you can't get away from me." It kept repeating. Some of the things I couldn't make out."
- "Once I heard a man's voice in my right ear say, 'This is your subconscious speaking to you.'"

One wonders if this last example could be counted as evidence in support of the "unconscious mind theory," or if, instead, the voice was that of a mischievous spirit who was out to deceive.

As with SP sufferers, the voices of schizophrenic are usually localized. They call from all directions, says Jaynes, but very rarely do they come from directly in front of the patient. This, by the way, is also true of the auditory hallucinations I've heard – not once have I heard a voice emanate from directly in front of me. Interestingly, Cheyne mentions that the visual hallucinations of SP sufferers, as well as the sensed presence, "are almost out of sight, on the periphery of vision or obscured by ambient shadows." Reading these words, one is immediately reminded of the voices heard by schizophrenics. In both cases, there is a hidden quality to the hallucinations, as though whatever is behind them doesn't wish to reveal itself completely.

According to Jaynes, the voices of schizophrenics appear to emanate from many different objects, substances, and places. They might seem to come from walls, for example, from the roof, from near or far, or from parts of the body. In some instances, moreover, as one patient put it, "they assume the nature of all those objects through which they speak – whether they speak out of walls, or from ventilator, or in the woods and fields."

Some patients, says Jaynes, associate the good, consoling voices with the upper right, and the bad ones from below and to the left. In many religions and cultures throughout the world, we find that the left side of the body, particularly the left hand, is associated with evil, and the right with good. According to Gooch in *The Origins of Psychic Phenomena*, which features a chapter on the psychic significance of left-handedness, "Muslims believe that both prophets and diviners are inspired by familiars; but whereas the former, who wear white, hear the words of their invisible companions at their right ear, the latter, who wear black, receive their instruction in the left ear." In Western occultism, reference is often made to the "left-hand path" and the "right-hand path." The latter is God-centered and involves strict observance of moral codes; the former is self-centered and "morally loose."

I think most SP sufferers will find that the sinister voice or noise that accompanies their worst and most frightening attacks is heard in their left ear, or on the left side of the body, as opposed to the right. This has been the case in my experience, anyway. The left-ear, of course, is controlled by the right side of the brain – the emotional, creative side – which as we know is thought by some to be the seat of the unconscious mind.

In 1992, as part of his research for *Muses, Madmen and Prophets*, Smith interviewed a schizophrenic outpatient at a New York psychiatric hospital, a man in his late-thirties called Richard K. At the age of fourteen, while sitting in class one day, Richard heard laughter and mumbling coming from somewhere *behind and to the left of him*. A shy, awkward boy, who was often made fun of, Richard suddenly turned around, thinking he'd see a bully seated behind him. But none of his classmates had uttered a sound. They looked at him in silence and bewilderment. Experiences of this kind persisted and became more frequent. In the afternoons, while walking home from school, Richard would often hear a disembodied voice calling out his name from across the street. It had, he said, a slightly tinny quality, as though spoken through an old microphone.

Fearing that he'd lost his sanity, or was very close to doing so, Richard confided in his older brother, the only person he trusted. His brother told him he was not crazy but that other people would think he was and that he should not tell anyone else about the voices, otherwise, "they'll pump you full of Thorazine and lock you away forever." He took his brother's advice. When he entered high school, Richard's situation became even worse. He was teased mercilessly. "High school," he said, "messed up my voices bad." A new voice emerged at this point, different in quality to the other one. It could be heard internally rather than externally, and possessed a specific tone. He imagined the source of the voice to be a tall man in a dark suit, wearing a ring, and called it "the Executive." The voice offered him advice, gave him a sense of psychological security, and helped him manage his life.

Before long, however, the Executive began to attract a series of other voices – a kind of administration made up of various councils and such. There emerged, writes Smith, "a complex political structure inside Richard's head. First, there was the Troika, a three-member cabinet that advised the Executive on the daily strategy of conducting Richard's life. Next there was the Full-Movement Council, a legislative body comprised of several hundred members..." And so on and so forth. There even existed an "opposition leader," known as the "Anti-Executive," whose job was to undermine the executive's efforts. Although these additional voices *did* help organize the clutter in his mind, they proved overwhelmingly distracting, causing more harm than good. Sometimes they'd all speak at once, says Richard, sounding as if a "symphony of un-tuned instruments was playing very loudly inside my head."

Despite the presence of the voices and the fact that they tortured him daily, Richard managed to graduate from high school and also get married. But partly as a result of the voices, his marriage eventually came to an end. His wife found out about them when, one day, Richard said he heard them coming from a radio that was not switched on. When she realized that the voices existed only in Richard's head, her reaction was one of absolute terror. After suffering a psychotic episode, Richard was admitted to a mental hospital and prescribed antipsychotic medication.

In time his mental health improved, and he managed to gain employment as a caseworker. But the treatment he was given did not block out the voices completely. One voice appeared that was actually quite helpful, and which, he told Smith, he was glad his medication did not erase. It was different from all the others, he said. He described it to Smith as "like a sign. It is like an impression in my soul. I listen to the impression and I give words to it. I verbalize the impression...It is not easy to hear the voice. The universe that we live in screens it out, like a prism refracts light. And so what I hear is almost like prophecy itself." It was, he believed, the voice of God.

CHAPTER 13

Caught Between Heaven And Hell

O Rose, thou art sick.
The Invisible worm,
That flies in the night,
In the howling storm,

Has found out thy bed
Of Crimson joy:
And his dark secret love
Does thy life destroy.
– William Blake, "The Sick Rose, Songs of Experience," 1794

Clinical psychologist Wilson Van Dusen, formerly of the Mendocino State Hospital in California, spent sixteen years studying the nature of hallucinations and their effects, some of which he actually "talked to" by getting the patients to relate, as accurately as possible, what they were seeing and hearing. "In this way," he says, "I could hold long dialogues with a patient's hallucinations and record both my questions and their answers." Not all of the patients involved in his study were schizophrenic. Some of them were alcoholics. Others were brain damaged or senile. Van Dusen emphasizes that our common conception of the mentally ill is flawed. The majority of them, he says, are not "raving lunatics" as one might think. "Most of these people have become entangled in inner processes and simply fail to manage their lives well."

Although the patients he worked with suffered from hallucinations for a variety of different reasons, their experiences were remarkably similar, noted Van Dusen. Because the patients thought of their hallucinations as objectively real, he approached them as a phenomenologist. According to Jaynes in *The Origins of Consciousness*, "the voices a patient hears are more real than the doctor's voice." Jaynes includes the following humorous quote, given by a schizophrenic patient who was questioned by a doctor about the reality of his voices: "Yes, sir. I hear voices distinctly, even loudly; they interrupt us at this moment. It is more easy for me to listen to them than to you. I can more easily believe in their significance and actuality, and they do not ask questions."

As happened to the aforementioned Richard K., the hallucinations of Van Dusen's patients generally came on suddenly. In the majority of cases, instead of making a gradual entrance into the patient's life, as one would expect, the voices – and sometimes visions – appeared one day totally out of the blue. One man, for example, was riding on a bus when he heard a piercing scream. He had to plead with the voice to get it to quiet down. Another patients described how, while working alone in her garden one day, a friendly man approached her, and they started to chat. "Most patients," says Van Dusen, "were brought into somewhat sinister relationships [with their hallucinations]. Already estranged from society, they hopefully took up with these promising new friends who talked like kindly helpful people with great powers. Gradually they found their new friends were liars who were more and more critical and tormenting of them…"

According to Van Dusen, most patients learn to keep quiet about their experiences, knowing that others will think them deranged, when, for example, the patient suddenly realizes that no one else can see the CIA agent who's been following them around for weeks or hear the man's voice that's coming from the air vent. They might get by in this manner for a while, their friends and relatives none the wiser. Eventually, however, the truth comes to light, for who could maintain such a profound secret? What sometimes happens is that the patient's sanity will be doubted when they describe seeing or hearing something that is not a part of objective reality.

The visual hallucinations of schizophrenics, like the voices, are experienced in such a manner as to appear fully real. One patient told Van Dusen of having been awakened at night by a group of Air Force officers "calling him to the service of his country." While sleepily getting dressed and ready to leave, the man suddenly noticed that the insignia they wore wasn't quite right and realized they were not to be trusted. He tried to punch one of the "officers" in the face but ended up injuring his hand, which passed straight through the figure and struck the wall behind it.

A female patient said she regularly saw President Gamal Abdel Nasser (a former president of Egypt) and had been doing so for many years. He would sometimes be seated in an empty chair in Van Dusen's office, she claimed. Van Dusen tried an experiment to test the patient's perception of the hallucination, passing his hand behind "the president" and down the back of the chair. The patient was unable to see the part of his hand that was behind the hallucination.

Van Dusen soon discovered that his patients' hallucinations were of two completely opposite types. One type, which was by far the most common, he termed the "lower order." The other he termed the "higher order." He refers to them, occasionally, as "lower order voices," and "higher order voices," even though the hallucinations may have been, depending on the patient, both auditory and visual in nature, just auditory, or just visual. "For reasons that puzzle me," he says, "some patients experience only auditory voices, some just visions, some a mix of these."

He compares lower order voices to "drunken bums at a bar who like to tease and torment just for the fun of it...They call the patient every conceivable name, suggest every lewd act, steal memories or ideas right out of consciousness, threaten death, and work on the patient's credibility in every way." They can even inflict "felt pain as a way of enforcing their power."

Van Dusen continues: "These hallucinations lie, cheat, deceive, pretend, threaten, etc. Dealing with them is like dealing with very mean drunks. Nothing pleases them. They see the negative side of everything. Catching them in a bold lie doesn't even embarrass them. Their main aim seems to be to live it up at the patient's expense. I asked one lower order man what his purposes were. He said, 'Fight, screw, win the world.' They zero in on every fault or guilt of the patient and play on it. *Their aim seems to be to take over the patient and live through him as they please*" (my emphasis).

The lower order, he says, appeared to occupy a region of the patient's mind but not their entire mind. It would not be inaccurate to term them "mind parasites." Van Dusen mentions that these "other people" are able to experience what the patient experiences and can see what they see. For instance, he says, "If I showed a patient an ink blot, the voice could see it too." Van Dusen used this to his advantage, administering psychological tests not only to the patients but to their voices as well. Apparently, "most hallucinations looked much sicker than the patient."

Much like lower astral entities that present themselves at séances, the lower order voices "never have a personal identity though they accept most identities given them" and "either conceal or have no awareness of personal memories." Van Dusen adds: "Though they claim to be separate identities they will reveal no detail which might help to trace them as separate individuals...When identified as some friend known to the patient they can assume this voice quality perfectly."

Van Dusen first details his findings in a chapter titled "The Presence of Spirits in Madness" in his book *The Presence of Other Worlds* (1974), and although he makes no specific reference to "lower astral entities" he does mention "evil spirits" – that is, evil spirits as described by the Swedish religious mystic Emanuel Swedenborg (1688-1772), who claimed to have encountered such beings, and to have journey to heaven and hell. Very much a shaman, Swedenborg used the hypnagogic state as a portal to the "spirit realm." There are, says Van Dusen, a large number of uncanny similarities between the lower order voices of his patients and the evil spirits described by Swedenborg. I will explain this aspect of his research in a moment.

The boastful lower order voices claimed to possess great powers, such as that of ESP and precognition. But, more often than not, their words rang hollow. Their intention was to scare and unnerve the patient, by insisting, for instance, that they would die on a particular day. Whenever she played cards, complained one woman, voices would ruin the game by reading off her opponent's cards. This became so annoying that she stopped playing cards altogether. "Unfortunately," writes Van Dusen, "ESP just seems to frighten the patient further. I've not heard of any instance where a patient could make any constructive use of it."

Only when the patient is asleep do the voices stop speaking, says Van Dusen. As soon as they wake up, the voices start again. Just to be spiteful, they will sometimes keep a patient up by talking non-stop. Most patients will go to great lengths to rid themselves of the voices, some by keeping crosses around them, others by praying or by changing their diet. But none of these measures work. Van Dusen notes that ataractic drugs, such as Thorazine, don't necessarily stop the voices, "but they do lessen the patient's reaction to them." Attempts to ignore the voices and visions don't help either. One patient is quoted as saying, "How do you feel when you go to take a leak and find someone else's hand on your cock? There is just no privacy anywhere!"

Van Dusen describes how one of his female patients heard a voice claiming to be Jesus Christ. As can sometimes happen with patients and their voices, the two of them had become lovers. The voice boasted that it possessed psychic powers, saying it could read people's minds. Van Dusen decided to put it to the test, writing numbers on a hidden piece of paper and asking the voice to psychically read them. Not once was the voice successful. The patient soon concluded that the voice was crazy, deluded, and needed help, so she tried to counsel it. "He seemed to come to his senses gradually and left the woman," writes Van Dusen. "Some patients who had led rather immoral lives found their critical voices gradually came down in volume and left as they vigorously studied the Bible and led a very moral life."

Van Dusen then states: "Apparently it's quite possible for a person to have sexual intercourse with hallucinations. One woman described it as being more inward and much nicer than having a real man." The overwhelming significance of these words cannot have escaped the reader's attention. It's possible, as I've said, for a person to have sexual intercourse with a spirit, as many an SP sufferer and hypnagogic experimenter knows. I cannot overemphasize the realistic nature of these encounters. Here, again, are those words of Gooch's: "I can only say that the experience is totally satisfying...From some points of view the sex is actually more satisfying than that with a real woman..." People who have had these experiences – and I am one of them – all say exactly the same thing: that "spirit sex" is more fulfilling than "real sex." One could classify the former as "soul sex" as it takes place on an astral level.

What we have here is a direct connection between the experiences of SP sufferers, hypnagogic experimenters, and schizophrenics. If, as the evidence seems to indicate, the SP sufferer and the hypnagogic experimenter are able to have sex with spirits, and also hear the voices of spirits, and considering that schizophrenics also hear voices and are able to have sexual intercourse with their hallucinations, would it not be unreasonable to suppose that schizophrenia is a form of spirit possession? So as not to arrive at a premature conclusion on the matter, let us examine the rest of Van Dusen's findings.

According to Van Dusen, the lower order voices were difficult to work with and relate to "because of their disdain for me as well as the patient." That they had "a persistent will to destroy the patient" could not be denied. Van Dusen describes the case of a man who, for ten days, heard voices arguing with each other as to how they should kill him. "They had a gun – he could hear its hammer fall – a hangman's rope, a flame for burning, etc. This conviction is experienced by many alcoholics who finally kill themselves to get it over with." The lower order voices, which sometimes referred to themselves as demons or beings from hell, all despised religion and would even interfere with the patients' religious practices.

Many patients claimed that the voices were trying to possess a part of their body or had already managed to do so. Apparently one voice managed to gain control of a patient's eye, and it actually went visibly out of alignment. They also tried to possess people's ears; when successful, the patient would become hard of hearing. Van Dusen was also aware of cases in which the patient's genitals had been possessed. Most startling of all, however, the voices were sometimes able to use the patient as a medium –

or, in Van Dusen's words, "seize the tongue and speak through the person."

Van Dusen found that the process of possession was a gradual one, with more and more of the patient being taken over as time when on. Some of the very psychotic patients behaved as if they had become almost completely possessed. Van Dusen writes: "I recall examining one man who professed to being moral and upright. In a few minutes the dirtiest talk would come from his mouth, mostly about assholes. I would remind him of his morality. Yes, yes, he would say, he was always careful to think clean thoughts. In the next minute he rambled on about menstrual cloths. It looked as if he was possessed and there was just a fragment of the original man present."

Perhaps there's some truth to the Christian belief in a heaven and hell – the former being populated by angels, and the other, by demons – with mankind trapped in the middle, between the two extremes. Each choice we make seems to lead us in either one of these directions. Do we choose to act selfishly or altruistically? Do we choose to listen to our conscience, or to the demon perched on our left shoulder? Or maybe a little of both? Many of us feel, on some level, that we're caught between heaven and hell – metaphorically speaking, of course. But schizophrenics feel this way on a literal level, and, as we know, they even see beings whom they take to be angels and demons. The "demons," of course, are what Van Dusen calls lower order voices.

Let us now move on to the "angels."

The reader may recall Daniel Smith's interview with the schizophrenic patient Richard K., and how Richard mentioned hearing "the voice of God," which he described as "like an impression in my soul." This is a beautiful description of what Van Dusen came to refer to as the "higher order." These "voices," he discovered, were in complete contrast to the lower order voices and were quite rare, making up a fifth or less of the patient's experiences. As though arising from a "superconscious" level of mind (or perhaps because they were a product of, or communicated through, the right brain), the higher order was able to think in "something like universal ideas" and in ways that were "richer and more complex than the patient's own mode of thought," reminding Van Dusen of Carl Jung's archetypes. Only rarely did the higher order use words to communicate, "whereas the lower order can talk endlessly." Van Dusen compares the lower order to Freud's Id. "In general," he says, "the higher order is richer than the patient's normal experience, respectful of his freedom, helpful, instructive, supportive, highly symbolic and religious."

Van Dusen mentions how one of his male patients, who kept hearing voices arguing with each other as to how they should murder him, was visited at night by a bright light, similar in appearance to the sun. The entity, which respected the man's freedom "and would withdraw if it frightened him," took him on a spiritual journey of sorts, whereby "he entered a world of powerful numinous experiences." During one part of the journey, the man found himself at the end of a long corridor, facing a large door, behind which "raged the powers of hell." He was tempted to open the door and was about to do so when a Christ-like figure appeared, telling him telepathically to take a more suitable course of action. The entity encouraged the man to "follow him into other experiences which were therapeutic to him." Some of these experiences were frightening, yet ultimately beneficial to the man. (I am reminded of the first few lines of Rainer Maria Rilke's poem *The Second Elegy*: "Every Angel is terrible. Still, though, alas! I invoke you, almost deadly birds of the soul, knowing what you are.")

The patient, a high school-educated gas pipefitter, had encounters with other higher order beings, one of whom was an attractive, sprightly little woman who referred to herself as "An Emanation of the Feminine Aspect of the Divine." Sweet, friendly, and respectful, she befriended the patient because she wished to cheer him up and would play all kinds of entertaining jokes. The patient had asked her if she wished to have a sexual relationship with him, but she politely refused, saying it wouldn't be appropriate. Van Dusen was able to communicate with the entity by getting her to nod yes or no in response to his questions. (He, of course, was unable to see or hear her; only the patient could.) Naturally, Van Dusen treated the "woman" as though she were more than just a product of the patient's imagination: "Whenever I or the patient said something very right, she would come over to us and hand us her panties."

The entity possessed a remarkable knowledge of all things spiritual and religious, communicating most of her ideas in the form of universal symbols, some of which pertained to Greek myths. She also appeared to have some degree of ESP and, unlike those of the lower order, was genuinely able to read people's minds, including Van Dusen's. He once asked her to symbolize his mood, all the while trying not to let on how he actually felt. The image she used was that of a limp penis – "a surprisingly accurate representation of my feelings." When he asked the patient much the same question – how he felt emotionally, that is – the response he received was: "Okay, just average, I guess." Van Dusen stresses the point that the entity was far wiser, knowledgeable, and intelligent than the patient, and that much of what she said went straight over the patient's head and, at times, his own.

Van Dusen was obviously deeply impressed by the entity (what most other psychologists would probably call "a meaningless hallucination"), describing her, quite flatteringly, as "the most gifted person in the area of religion I've ever known." He asked her all manner of religious questions, and the answers he received were most enlightening. "She was entirely unlike talking to earthly theologians who call on history to prove a point," says Van Dusen. "She knew the depth of my understanding and led gently into very human allusions that reflected a profound understanding of history."

The purpose of the lower order, according to the higher order, is to make the patient aware of their weaknesses and faults – but neither in a helpful nor a constructive way. Such voices, as I've said, can drive a person to suicide, especially if that person believes what they say. A little bit of criticism can be helpful, but if your are called "a worthless piece of shit" about fifty times a day, it's bound to have a detrimental effect on your self-esteem and overall mental health, to say the least. Most of us have no idea of the pain and torture that auditory hallucinations cause. Fortunately, discovered Van Dusen, the higher order proved to have some power over the lower order, "but not enough to give peace of mind to most patients."

To gain a proper understanding of Van Dusen's research, it's necessary that I mention a little about Swedenborg, that great Swedish shaman of the 18th century, who, according to Van Dusen, "probably explored the hypnagogic state more than any other man has ever done before or since." According to Van Dusen in *The Presence of Other Worlds*, "all Swedenborg's observations on the effect of evil spirits entering man's consciousness conform to my findings." Not only was Swedenborg an important religious figure (more so after his death than before it), he was also a scientist, inventor, and philosopher. It was not until the age of fifty-six that Swedenborg became interested in spiritual and religious matters, having undergone what can only be described as a "spiritual awakening," whereby he experienced strange dreams and visions, some of them quite frightening and confronting. According to Swedenborg, the Lord had "opened his eyes," permitting him access to heaven and hell; allowing him, moreover, to meet and converse with angels, demons, and other spirits. Swedenborg further claimed that the Lord had appointed him to write a heavenly doctrine, and that its purpose was to reform Christianity.

Born in the city of Stockholm in 1688, Swedenborg was raised in a highly religious environment. His father, Jesper Swedberg, was professor of theology at Uppsala University and also the Bishop of Skara. His mother, Sara Behm, a kind and gentle soul, died when he was eight years old. (The change of the family name from Swedberg to Swedenborg came about through Jesper's doing.) Something of a Christian mystic, as Swedenborg would also become, Jesper believed in the existence of angels and spirits. Such beings, he felt, were able to influence humanity on an everyday level. He also believed that a Christian should seek communion with God rather than rely on faith alone. The family was fond of discussing religious matters, even around the dinner table, and it's fair to say that Jesper's unconventional religious beliefs had a strong influence on the young Swedenborg. "I was constantly engaged in thought upon God, salvation, and the spiritual sufferings of men..." he once wrote, recalling his youth.

After completing his studies at Upsala University in 1709, Swedenborg traveled extensively throughout Europe, eventually reaching London where he continued his education, studying physics, mechanics, mathematics, politics, and a plethora of other subjects. "In an age when relatively few men became really learned, Emanuel Swedenborg spent the first thirty-five years of his life in a massive program of formal and self-directed education," explains Sig Synnestvedt in *The Essential Swedenborg*.

A man of astounding intellect, there seemed to be almost nothing his mind couldn't grasp. He was an accomplished linguist, speaking nine languages fluently, but ironically he suffered from a speech impediment. As a young man, Swedenborg dreamed of becoming a great scientist and inventor. He knew, in fact, that he was destined to achieve greatness. Two of his inventions include a submarine and a flying machine.

According to Colin Wilson in his tour de force *The Occult*, Swedenborg "was an intensely frustrated man," and also "highly sexed," who "escaped his frustrations through hard work." Highly sexed or not, Swedenborg remained a bachelor his whole life. He apparently fell in love with a Miss Pelham, who accepted him at first, only to break off the engagement soon afterwards. This incident, says Wilson, "must have been a blow on every level: of pride of emotion and of purely masculine sexuality." He apparently tried to marry a second time, but was also rejected.

Wilson points out that Swedenborg possessed an enormous amount of energy and drive, and indeed this cannot be denied. At age twenty-eight, King Charles XII of Sweden appointed him Extraordinary Assessor of the Royal College of Mines. In 1713, Charles XII asked him to devise a way to transport five ships across fifteen miles of dry land – a task he completed in seven weeks. His career as assessor involved a wide range of tough responsibilities. He had to inspect mines, render detailed reports on the quality and amount of mined ore, and also solve various personnel and administrative problems.

Not only was Swedenborg involved in scientific and engineering matters, but political ones also, and he served at the House of Nobles for some fifty years. In 1747, he resigned his position as a member of the Board of Mines, stating that he wished to dedicate his time to other interests. For several years he edited a scientific journal called *Daedalus*, the first of its kind to be published in Sweden. He also wrote books on scientific subjects, including algebra, astronomy, minerals, economics, the tides, metallurgy, salt mining, biology, and astronomy. Many of his scientific ideas and discoveries were far ahead of their time and remained little appreciated by his contemporaries. Most notably, he is credited with supplying the first accurate understanding of the importance of the cerebral cortex. His metallurgical findings, involving the treatment of iron, copper and brass, were also of great importance.

During the next phase of his life, from about 1720 to 1745, Swedenborg focused his attention on matters of a philosophic nature – cosmology in particular, as well as the nature of the human soul. The amount of material he wrote on these subjects is astounding. Perhaps his most important effort is a three-volume work entitled *Philosophical and Mineralogical Works*. Other works include *The Economy of the Animal Kingdom*, *The Brain*, *The Senses*, and *The Organs of Generation*, not all of which were published during his lifetime.

Swedenborg's aforementioned "spiritual awakening" occurred around 1744, when he began to have visions and strange dreams, some of them frightening, others exhilarating. He feared he was losing his sanity. He kept quiet about these experiences but fortunately wrote them down, recording them in his *Journal of Dreams* and *Journal of Travel*. The first work in particular is still of much interests to psychologists. In one horrifying nightmare he was caught in the wheel of a huge machine. In another, he felt between a woman's legs, only to find her vagina full of teeth.

It's interesting to note that part of the initiatory process of becoming a shaman involves a period of "spiritual sickness," whereby the shaman-to-be sufferers from visions and frightening dreams, and sometimes develops a fever. If he comes out alive, so to speak, he develops healing powers and begins his formal training as a shaman. To pass such a "test," one must battle one's inner and outer demons, and find a source of strength within oneself. Only the strongest souls become shamans. Other less fortunate individuals end up losing their grip on reality; fortunately, Swedenborg did not.

In 1745, while dining alone at a London inn, Swedenborg had a vision in which the room grew dark and a spirit spoke to him. He was told to fulfill an important mission for God – a mission that would involve acting as a channel of sorts. He believed that God had called him to bring a new revelation to the world; from that point on, he began writing about theological matters, pouring out page after page of divine revelation. His magnum opus, *Arcana Coelestia* (*Heavenly Secrets*), which is more than 7,000 pages long, is a spiritual interpretation of the books of Genesis and Exodus, and formed the basis of his numerous other theological works, which include *Heaven and Hell*, *The New Jerusalem and its Heavenly Doctrine*, *Doctrine of the Lord*, *Apocalypse Revealed,* and *True Christian Religion.* Swedenborg believed that the teachings and events in the bible are not to be interpreted in a literal fashion but contain deeper meanings of which most people are unaware. In his opinion, for example, The Exodus from Egypt is a symbolic description of the process of spiritual growth that we all undergo and the many struggles we encounter during this journey.

Having been granted access to the "spirit realm," Swedenborg was able to gain information clairvoyantly. On one occasion, while dining with friends in the city of Gothenburg, he suddenly became distressed. A fire, he said, had broken out in Stockholm, and his house was in danger of burning down. Later that night, he exclaimed: "Thank God! The fire is extinguished the third door from my house!" Stockholm was located 300 miles away, and news of the fire did not reach the people of Gothenberg until well after Swedenborg had "seen" the event in his mind. The details he had given of the incident proved to be correct. This unintentional demonstration of "second sight" generated some fame for Swedenborg, as did a number of other remarkable incidents.

On another occasion, after hearing of his alleged ability to communicate with spirits, the widow of a Dutch ambassador, Mme. de Marteville, asked Swedenborg if he could contact her dead husband regarding a certain financial matter. A silversmith had sent her a large bill for some work that he had done for her husband, yet she was sure that he had paid it prior to his death. She thought the receipt was located somewhere in the house, but she couldn't find it. If, said Swedenborg, he saw her husband while next in the "spirit realm," he would try and solve the problem.

A few days later, Swedenborg had some interesting news to report. He had encountered her husband, who told him that he would tell her where the receipt was located. About a week later, the woman saw her husband in a dream. He led her to a desk in the house, telling her to look behind a particular drawer – and indeed the receipt was found to be located in this exact spot. She also found a diamond hairpin that had gone missing. The following morning, Swedenborg paid another visit to the woman, and before she had the chance to tell him about her dream, he explained that he had encountered her husband a second time. They had been talking last night, he said, but the conversation had to be cut short when the dead ambassador explained that he needed to tell his wife about the missing receipt.

In 1761, Queen Lovisa Ulrika asked Swedenborg if he would communicate with her late brother, Augustus William, Prince Royal of Prussia. To this he agreed, visiting her again a couple of days later at court while her ladies of honor surrounded her. Count Hopken, one of Swedenborg's contemporaries, relates the rest of this story: "Swedenborg not only greeted her [the Queen] from her brother, but also gave her his apologies for not having answered her last letter; he also wished to do so now through Swedenborg; which he accordingly did. The Queen was greatly overcome, and said: 'No one but God knows this secret.'"

Swedenborg is considered to have been a kind and modest man, and was greatly admired by those who knew him. Not once did he try and convert people to his beliefs, and in no way did he consider himself superior to anyone else, despite the fact that he'd been specially chosen by God to fulfill a religious mission – or so he believed. In his book *Channeling*, Jon Klimo describes him as "one of the true giants of channeling literature." That Swedenborg was a channeler, who penned his material in a state of trance, perhaps by means of automatic writing, might help explain his ability to write so prolifically.

When, nearing the end of his life, Swedenborg was asked to comment on the truth or falsity of the new revelation he had communicated through his writings, he replied: "As truly as you see me before your eyes, so true is everything that I have written; and I could have said more had it been permitted. When you enter eternity you will see everything, and then you and I shall have much to talk about."

As regards evil spirits and their influence on mankind, Swedenborg's views are strikingly similar to those of spiritist doctrine. They exert, be believed, a profound influence on the way we think and act but normally remain unaware of our existence, just as we normally remain unaware of theirs because a kind of barrier exists between them and our consciousness.

When, in some rare cases, this barrier is penetrated, all sorts of trouble results, including the hearing of annoying spirit voices. At the present day, writes Swedenborg in *Heaven and Hell*, "to talk with spirits is rarely granted because it is dangerous."

Swedenborg explains the reason why: "For then the spirits know, what otherwise they do not know, that they are with man, and evil spirits are such that they hold man in deadly hatred, and desire nothing more than to destroy him both soul and body, which indeed happens with those who have so indulged themselves in fantasies as to have separated from themselves the enjoyments proper to the natural man. Some also who lead a solitary life sometimes hear spirits talking with them, and without danger; but that the spirits with them may not know that they are with man they are at intervals removed by the Lord; for most spirits are not aware that any other world than that in which they live is possible, and therefore are unaware that there are men anywhere else. This is why man on his part is not permitted to speak with them, for if he did they would know."

As Van Dusen points out, Swedenborg came up with a remarkably accurate description of what we nowadays call schizophrenia, defining such people as "those who have so indulged themselves in fantasies as to have separated from themselves the enjoyments proper to the natural man." A modern definition of the term, as given by the *Penguin English Dictionary*, is not all that dissimilar: "Any of several mental disorders characterised by loss of contact with reality and disintegration of personality…" Eugen Bleuler was the first psychiatrist to clearly delineate schizophrenia – a term that he coined. This occurred in 1911, about 150 years after the death of Swedenborg, whose understanding of mental illness was clearly ahead of its time.

Swedenborg believed that the good and bad spirits that populate the spirit realm work through us, much in the same way that electricity works through the various components of a circuit. He saw the universe as consisting of many levels, ordered in a hierarchical nature, with both a positive and a negative side, all of it operating in total balance. At the top of Swedenborg's "model" is the Lord. The Lord acts through three levels of heaven – or, more specifically, the angels that inhabit these three individual levels – one situated above the other, as it were. These three heavens, says Swedenborg, "constitute three expanses," which "communicate with each other by the Divine influx from the Lord out of the sun of the spiritual world." Below these exist three levels of hell, "between which in like manner there is provided a communication by means of an influx through the heavens from the Lord."

Existing between these two great hierarchies is man, who is the sum total of the influx that emanates from heaven and the influx that emanates from hell. Both of these realms act into man equally. "So long as man is living in the world," says Swedenborg, "he is kept and walks midway between heaven and hell, and there he is in spiritual equilibrium, which is his freedom of choice...Because man is midway between these two opposites, and at the same time in spiritual equilibrium, he is able to choose, adopt, and appropriate to himself from freedom either the one or the other. If he chooses evil and falsity he connects himself with hell; if he chooses good and truth he connects himself with heaven."

Swedenborg goes so far as to say that spirits are adjoined to one's spirit but in such a way that one is not aware of them, and vice versa. Van Dusen explains this in modern terms, saying that "spirits are in the unconscious." Because spirits think spiritually and man naturally, a corresponding effect takes place. Spirits exert an influence on our thoughts and feelings, but we don't realize it – or at least most of us don't, schizophrenics being an exception. We think such thoughts and feelings are our own. We exist in our reality and they exist in theirs, and we each go about our own separate business. Nonetheless, we act together.

Good spirits, or angels, says Swedenborg, dwell in the most interior aspects of one's mind (in what Van Dusen refers to as one's "loves, affections, or ends"), while evil spirits dwell in an even lower but still unconscious level of one's mind – one's personal memory. "These spirits," says Swedenborg, "have no knowledge whatever that they are with man; but when they are with him they believe that all things of his memory and thought are their own." Swedenborg thought that we each have four spirits with us during our lives – two good and two evil. The good spirits act as our intermediaries with heaven, and the evil spirits act as our intermediaries with hell. Were they not to exist, these "links in the cosmic chain," we would have no connection with either realm.

As mentioned previously, the "barrier of awareness" preventing spirits from realizing that they exist alongside mankind is at risk of being penetrated when one withdraws from the world into one's own head. Swedenborg, of course, was able to "lift" this barrier at will as a result of entering a sustained hypnagogic state. And, just as importantly, he was able to seal the barrier closed when need be. Swedenborg believed, perhaps simplistically, that God was the one preventing him from being harmed by evil spirits; that he was able to enter hell, and even have his body temporarily possessed by demons, because God was his guide and protector. He further believed that he was required to undertake these journeys, even though some of them were frightening and unpleasant, so as to bring back important knowledge that would benefit mankind.

Once the barrier is penetrated, says Swedenborg, evil spirits suddenly realize that they exist independently of man. They then begin to communicate with him, and in such a way as to cause him the maximum amount of suffering and torment as they can. "For evil spirits, being conjoined with hell, desire nothing so much as to destroy man, not alone his soul, that is, his faith and love, but also his body."

When due to their love of "mundane and earthly things" evil spirits "enter into man" and "obsess him," says Swedenborg, they invade his memory, consequently losing their own personal memory. This process is a kind of death for the spirit because it forgets who it is, yet retains its more interior aspects. Assuming this is true, it might help explain why the lower order voices, although they acted as separate individuals, were unable to reveal "even a trace of personal identity, nor even a name." Van Dusen speculates that extreme cases of schizophrenia may be instances in which the spirit (or spirits) troubling the patient has taken on more of their own memory. This could apply, he says, to those patients he studied who came across as victims of "spirit possession." Swedenborg writes: "For were spirits to retain their corporeal memory, they would so far obsess man, that he would have no more self-control or be in the enjoyment of his life, than one actually obsessed."

Swedenborg's teachings seem to suggest that "mind parasites," or evil spirits, influence us all, but because they normally exist in a "deactivated" state, we remain unaware of their existence. Only if they happen to "wake up" can they noticeably harm us. Fortunately, though, we're also in "communication" with benevolent spirits, whose influence brings a much needed balance to the process.

As for why the lower order proves more common than the higher order, Van Dusen found that Swedenborg's teachings provide a logical and satisfying answer. Angels, according to Swedenborg, possess the very interior of man, while their influx "takes place in accordance with the man's affections, which they gently lead and bend to good, and do not break, the very influx being tacit and scarcely perceptible, for it flows into the interiors, and continually acts by means of freedom." On the other hand, the influence of evil spirits is more explicit and noticeable.

Van Dusen was unable to dismiss his patients' hallucinations as creations of the unconscious mind – an explanation, he says, that fails to explain all the facts. According to him, it's just as likely – perhaps more likely – that "spiritual forces" existing independently of the patient are responsible, exactly as Swedenborg claimed. If the voices were "merely the patient's unconscious coming forth," then why is it, he asks, that the majority of lower order voices were found to have an extreme hatred of religion? "I would have no reason to expect them to be particularly for or against religion," he explains. "Yet the lower order can be counted on to give its most scurrilous comment to any suggestion of religion. They either totally deny any afterlife or oppose God and all religious practices." One is reminded of the Enfield poltergeist's extremely negative reaction to anything of a religious nature. Do all bad spirits have a hatred of religion?

Also, why were the patients' hallucinations all so similar? As Wilson points out in his book *Afterlife*, in a chapter concerning Van Dusen's research, "one might expect to find as many different types of hallucinations as there are people. For example, one might expect vets to have hallucinations that claim to be talking animals, engineers to be tormented by talking machines," and so on.

Although Van Dusen's leanings are towards the "spirit hypothesis," he gives the "unconscious mind theory" some credit too. "It might be that it is not either/or," he says. "If these two views should be the same thing then my brothers may be my keeper and I theirs simultaneously." It's interesting to note that the same argument comes up in regards to mediumship, in that neither one possibility fits the facts perfectly; the answer, it would seem, is a combination of both.

What's so startling about Van Dusen's study is that his findings are almost identical to those obtained by Swedenborg – who, remember, wasn't a madman at all but a perfectly competent member of society. He certainly did not suffer from any kind of mental illness, least of all schizophrenia. Everyone who knew him attested to his sanity. Even when he began to converse with spirits on a daily basis, his life was a productive and successful one. It should be mentioned, furthermore, that Van Dusen established his findings years before he had studied Swedenborg's position on the matter. "I'm inclined to believe that Swedenborg and I are dealing with the same matter," he says, and that "we are looking at a process which transcends cultures and remains stable over time."

Van Dusen admits that his findings, as well as Swedenborg's, have deeply unsettling implications, not only because they seem to suggest that spirit possession is a very real possibility, but because they raise questions about free will. He mentions, for instance, that one is able to undergo experiences similar to Swedenborg's as a result of entering the hypnagogic state. "With the experience of alien forces in this state," he says, "one comes to recognize their operation on impulsive thoughts in normal consciousness." How many of our thoughts, I wonder, are not really our own? Are our minds being influenced by spirits almost constantly and to an extent beyond our wildest imaginings?

Van Dusen explores these same questions, when he writes: "It is curious to reflect that, as Swedenborg has indicated, our lives may be the little free space at the confluence of giant higher and lower spiritual hierarchies. *It may well be this confluence is normal and only seems abnormal, as in hallucinations, when we become aware of being met by these forces* [my emphasis]. There is some kind of lesson in this – man freely poised between good and evil, under the influence of cosmic forces he usually doesn't know exist. Man, thinking he chooses, may be the resultant of other forces."

This brings us back to the subject of mediumship. According to Chico Xavier's *In the Domain of Mediumship*, which was mentioned in a previous chapter, everything in existence is a medium of sorts. "The farmer is the medium of the harvest, the plant is the medium of the fruit…We give and receive everywhere, filtering the resources that surround us and modeling them according to our abilities." These words add new meaning to Swedenborg's philosophy, for it could be said that we are all "mediums" for the good and evil spirits that we attract – or, in a collective sense, mankind is a medium for good and evil spiritual forces.

But although everyone is a medium, not everyone is a "conscious medium." According to *The Mediums' Book*, if a medium were to begin receiving evil spirit communications, or if negative manifestations such as poltergeist distubances began around them, this would indicate that the medium is under an evil influence. However, the book continues, "*this influence would affect him whether he were a medium or not, and whether he believed in Spiritism or whether he did not. Medianimity gives a man the means of assuring himself in regard to the nature of the spirits who act upon him, and of opposing them if they are evil*" (my emphasis). In other words, mediumship equals awareness.

When we consider the fact that some SP attacks are possible attempts at possession by discarnate entities, and that, as Van Dusen's study demonstrates, some schizophrenics may be advanced victims of spirit possession, it's perhaps no coincidence that the onset of both conditions occurs at about the same age – that is, from late adolescence to early adulthood. This, as an author friend of mine pointed out, could well mean that some people start off as SP sufferers but, unable to defend themselves psychically, end up getting completely possessed by their discarnate attackers, only to be diagnosed eventually as schizophrenic. Shamans-to-be, as we know, undergo a period of "spiritual sickness" during which they are possessed by spirits, their ability to cope with the experience being a kind of test; failure, presumably, would result in the development of severe mental illness.

In two possible spirit possession cases examined in earlier chapters, whereby the victim had been diagnosed with schizophrenia, either the death of a loved one played some role – as in Mary's case – or the individual's troubles began shortly after they started dabbling in mediumship and "spirit communications," as in Roger's case. The likely influence of nefarious spirits in the lives of these individuals cannot be ignored, nor can the fact that they underwent SP-type experiences in both an internal and an external manner (although one must treat Mary's case with much more skepticism).

The relationship between SP and schizophrenia is, I admit, a difficult one to recognize – unless, as I have tried to do, one picks up on the finer details. The theory that SP attacks can result in the development of schizophrenia is just a short step away from the theory that these experiences can cause poltergeist disturbances. Both could be seen as different forms of spirit possession, of which there seems to be many, with some more severe than others.

CHAPTER 14

Spirits In The Brain

To further our understanding of the SP phenomenon, and hopefully get to the bottom of the mystery, we must now go back to the beginning, so to speak, by addressing a topic of indispensable importance – sleep. For mammals, sleep consists of two stages of brain activity – non-rapid eye movement (NREM) and rapid eye movement (REM). The latter is associated with dreaming, the former is not. These two periods alternate throughout the night with the REM stage getting progressively longer. This explains why dreams are more likely to occur towards the end of sleep.

During NREM sleep, one's heartbeat and breathing remain relatively uniform, and movement is possible. NREM sleepers will toss and turn in bed. They might also sleep walk and sleep talk. Dreaming is rare during this stage. An EEG recording of someone in NREM sleep will usually exhibit delta waves, which are very low in frequency, varying from between one to four hertz (cycles per second). (An electroencephalograph, or EEG, is an instrument used for detecting and recording the electrical activity of the brain.) NREM sleep allows the body to repair and regenerate tissue, build bone and muscle, and strengthen the immune system.

REM sleep, as the name implies, is characterized by rapid movement of the eyes. We undergo about four or five periods of REM sleep a night: the first lasts about ten minutes, while the final one lasts about an hour. Altogether, these REM stages occupy about twenty to twenty-five percent of our total sleep time. REM sleep is marked by extensive physiological changes, including accelerated respiration, increased brain activity, muscle relaxation, and, of course, eye movement. During REM sleep, we exhibit a combination of beta and alpha brain wave activity – the same type of activity associated with the normal waking state.

When we are active and busy, and most likely concentrating, our brain will exhibit beta wave activity, which ranges in frequency from about twelve to thirty Hz. Were we to lie down on the couch, relax, and perhaps close our eyes, our brain wave activity would most likely slow down, shifting from a beta state to an alpha state, which ranges in frequency from eight to twelve Hz. The SP state is characterized by abundant alpha activity. Throughout the waking day, our brains will shift from one frequency to the other but staying predominately in the beta range. This makes sense because most of us spend our time being busy, while very few of us really know how to relax.

Our body becomes paralyzed during REM sleep to prevent us from "acting out" our dreams. The brain locks down muscles in the body by signaling the inhibition of muscular contraction. Inhibitor signals are transmitted by the nervous and endocrine systems. In some rare cases, you may wake up from REM sleep, yet these inhibitor signals will continue to be sent by mistake. The same thing can happen when you are entering wakefully into the REM state. In both instances, an SP episode may result.

When, during the SP state, you are lying in bed in a state of paralysis due to the activity of the nervous and endocrine systems, which continue transmitting inhibitor signals to our muscles, it's quite possible, say some researchers, that these same systems keep sending out signals that stimulate dreaming, resulting in a quasi-continuation of the dreaming state, even though you feel awake; thus your brain is flooded by images, sounds, and sensations that may be taken to be real but which are actually a product of the dreaming state.

It has been speculated, moreover, that the visual cortex may play a role in producing the visual "hallucinations" of SP sufferers. According to some researchers, SP may be caused by either an over-activation of the neural populations governing the sleep-on state or, more likely, an under-activation of those governing the sleep-off state. Lending credence to this theory is the fact that serotonin and adrenergic reuptake inhibitors (i.e. antidepressants) have been proven to alleviate the SP condition.

Although the brain is awake during the SP state, and you feel as if you are fully awake and alert, the brain nonetheless displays electrical activity typical of REM sleep, as shown by research carried out by Kazuhiko Fukuda of Fukushima University. In a series of experiments he and his colleagues conducted in a sleep laboratory, SP sufferers were hooked up to an EEG and roused suddenly at various times in the night, the aim being to trigger SP attacks. This method proved effective, and Fukuda was able to gain a clear understanding of what goes on inside the brain during the SP state.

Fukuda's experiments were replicated and improved upon by Japanese sleep researcher Dr. Tomoka Takeuchi. In his study, which was virtually identical to Fukuda's, SP attacks were artificially induced in individuals with a high incidence of SP. Meanwhile, their brain activity was recorded on an EEG. His work demonstrates, in the words of Sevilla, "that SP episodes, at least the ones triggered in a laboratory setting when researchers can actually correlate behavior, narratives, and electrophysiology, originate in a physiological state we more or less understand, and equally, in the self-aware creativity of these REM states."

What enables the SP sufferer, lucid dreamer, and OBE traveler to experience "other realities" is that the states of consciousness they enter – which are not that far removed in "frequency" – all involve some injection of awareness into the dreaming state. Therefore, to enter the "spirit realm," all one has to do is become aware during sleep – a task more difficult than it sounds.

Because, as mentioned, the brains of those undergoing SP attacks, although awake, nonetheless display electrical activity typical of REM sleep, some researchers such Cheyne believe that the "hallucinations" of SP sufferers share a biological kinship with dreaming, and that these experiences are basically an intrusion of REM activity into wakefulness. But Hufford disagrees, noting that "the specific contents of the experience...have not been explained...If they are related to ordinary dreams by the presence of REM physiology, why is their content so consistently the same without apparent regard for culture?" In Bruce Bower's article, *Night of the Crusher*, Hufford is quoted as saying: "I don't have a good explanation for these [SP] experiences."

So although scientists have gained some understanding of what occurs inside the brain during an SP attack and have even managed to artificially induce such experiences – though only to a very basic degree – they are still unable to explain what causes the complex "hallucinations" of SP sufferers – the sights, sounds, sensations, etc. Being an SP sufferer myself, I know for a fact that these "hallucinations" are in no way connected to the dream state and are not, in other words, a continuation of one's dreams.

Every single time I've had an SP attack featuring auditory hallucinations, for instance, and have been able to remember the dream preceding it, I've been aware of the fact that the two experiences were in no way related. This also applies to the visual hallucinations I've had, such as when I saw the "troll" sitting on my bed. I did not dream about this entity beforehand. I cannot overemphasize the fact that SP experiences, instead of being vague and dream-like, are extremely organized and lucid and do not in any way resemble dreams. In the latter, one's imagination takes over and almost anything can happen. SP experiences, on the other hand, tend to follow an expected pattern, with one episode being much like another.

Why, Hufford asks, are the "hallucinations" of SP sufferers, though separated in time and by culture, so remarkably similar? How does one explain such common sensations as being strangled, of having one's bed shaken back and forth, or of being grasped by the hand? The same can be said of the voices SP sufferers hear, which, in Cheyne's words, "are typically simple and direct." Why don't the messages of these voices vary all that much from SP sufferer to SP sufferer? And why – as shown in previous chapters – do people in haunted houses experience the same types of phenomena as SP sufferers?

Some researchers believe that the auditory hallucinations experienced by SP sufferers and others, including schizophrenics, can be explained in terms of abnormal temporal lobe activity. In the 1960s, Canadian neurologist Wilder Penfield discovered that electrical stimulation of the temporal lobes can, under certain conditions, induce auditory hallucinations in someone who's awake. In recent years, other researchers, most notably Canadian neuroscientist Dr. Michael Persinger, have carried out further experiments on the strange effects induced by artificial stimulation of the temporal lobes.

In Persinger's experiments, participants were made to wear helmets that targeted their temporal lobes with weak magnetic fields (similar in strength to those generated by a computer monitor). About 80 percent of the participants said they felt, or sensed, an unexplained presence in the room. Some of these experiences took on a highly spiritual nature, with participants claiming that they felt the presence of "God." SP sufferers, as we know, commonly report the experience of a "sensed presence."

In an article published in *New Scientists*, entitled "Alien Abduction – The Inside Story," Susan Blackmore describes the time she visited Persinger's lab at Laurentian University of Sudbury, Ontario, where she was administered his famous "EM treatment." She wrote: "I was wide awake throughout. Nothing seemed to happen for the first ten minutes or so. Instructed to describe aloud anything that happened, I felt under pressure to say something, anything. Then suddenly my doubts vanished. 'I'm swaying. It's like being on a hammock.' Then it felt for all the world as though two hands had grabbed my shoulders and were bodily yanking me upright. I knew I was still lying in the reclining chair, but someone, or something, was pulling me up.

"Something seemed to get hold of my leg and pull it, distort it, and drag it up the wall. It felt as though I had been stretched half way up to the ceiling. Then came the emotions. Totally out of the blue, but intensely and vividly, I suddenly felt angry – not just mildly cross but that clear-minded anger out of which you act...After perhaps ten seconds, it was gone. Later, it was replaced by an equally sudden attack of fear. I was terrified – of nothing in particular...I felt weak and disoriented for a couple of hours after coming out of the chamber."

Blackmore's artificially induced SP attack/alien abduction episode strikes me as interesting but not particular impressive. That she felt invisible hands pull at, and touch, her body, catches my attention more than any other detail, for as we know this experience is common to the SP phenomenon. That she underwent "a sudden attack of fear" is noteworthy too. But this seems to be where the similarities end.

The theory, as put forward by Persinger and others, that a significant number of paranormal, religious, and spiritual experiences, including alien abduction episodes, OBEs, as well as some elements of SP episodes, are caused by bursts of electrical activity in the temporal lobes of the brain due to the effects of EM radiation remains hard to accept. Firstly, the impressive results claimed by Persinger have proven difficult to replicate, and it would appear that much hype and exaggeration surrounded his research – and still does. His experimental methodology was a little flawed, in that many of his participants knew what to expect –a mind-boggling spiritual experience – and thus experienced what they expected, and perhaps hoped, to experience.

A group of Swedish researchers at Uppsala University (the same university that Swedenborg attended as a young man) attempted to replicate Persinger's results but under much stricter conditions. Unlike Persinger, they made use of a double-blind protocol, so that neither the participants nor the experimenters interacting with the participants had any idea who was being exposed to the magnetic fields. The results they obtained were less than impressive. Of those who reported strong spiritual experiences – a total of three – two of them belonged to the control group, as did eleven out of twenty-two who said they had undergone subtle experiences.

The researchers concluded that the magnetic fields had no discernable effects on the participants' brains; and therefore, what some of them experienced was most likely due to the placebo effect. But Persinger strongly disagrees, arguing that the Swedish group failed to replicate his work because they did not expose the participants to magnetic fields for a long enough period of time to produce an effect. Regarding these new findings, Blackmore is quoted as saying: "When I went to Persinger's lab and underwent his procedures I had the most extraordinary experiences I've ever had. I'll be surprised if it turns out to be a placebo effect." So it seems the jury's still out.

Also controversial is Persinger's Tectonic Strain Theory (TST). Explained simply, the theory states that a correlation exists between geomagnetic activity and paranormal experiences and events, particularly the sighting of UFOs. Strains within the Earth's crust near seismic faults produce strong electromagnetic (EM) fields, which, suggests Persinger, can not only produce bodies of light that resemble UFOs, but can also, as his laboratory experiments have demonstrated, affect one's temporal lobes, inducing hallucinations of alien beings and such. Like many a devoted skeptic of paranormal phenomena, Persinger argues that what one sees during such experiences, such as in alleged cases of alien abduction, are based on images from popular culture.

Anyone with even a superficial understanding of ufology and the alien abduction phenomenon would realize that Persinger's TST is really "pushing it." It might explain a very small number of UFO sightings, but that's about its limit. It certainly fails to explain those cases of alien abduction where abductees comes away with strange scoop-marks on their bodies, or where multiple and independent witnesses are involved, all of whom report seeing the same thing. I will address the alien abduction phenomenon in a later chapter – more specifically, the close encounter experiences of the famous abductee and author Whitley Strieber. Strieber's experiences demonstrate – as we will later find out – that not all cases of alien abduction can be explained as a result of SP, that they are, in fact, distinct phenomenon.

Were it possible for Persinger's "seismic EM fields" to induce hallucinations in certain people – thus giving them the impression that they'd had elaborate close encounter experiences, for example – would it not also be possible for people to be affected in the same way by the EM radiation emitted by common household appliances, such as television sets and hair dryers? The fact of the matter is that devices such as these – which are likely to emit *more* EM radiation than seismic events – do not stimulate our temporal lobes. After all, it's not as though we see aliens every time we switch on the hairdryer. We live in an environment polluted by EM radiation, yet very rarely do people report seeing UFOs and alien beings.

However, contends Persinger, it may be that the magnitude of EM fields is less of a significant factor than the particular temporal patterns they induce. For an EM field to have a noticeable effect on the brain, he says, and to therefore produce vivid hallucinations, it must have particular qualities. The critical feature of the EM fields used in his experimental work, he adds, "is that they are complex sequences of patterns containing information to which neurons and aggregates of neurons respond." This explains why they had a definite – though perhaps exaggerated – effect.

In an inventive attempt to determine if spiking EM fields and extremely low frequency sound waves (infrasound) can affect the brain in such a way as to create the illusion that a location is haunted, psychology professor Chris French of the Anomalistic Psychology Research Unit at Goldsmiths College, UK, together with a team of assistants, set up a "haunted" room in a London apartment, rigged with EM sources and infrasound generators. (Infrasound is so low in frequency that it cannot be heard by the human ear, and is known to induce feelings of fear and uneasiness.) All of the equipment – including twin coils that generated EM pulses of up to fifty microteslas, as well as a computer that was used to emit infrasound of 19.9 and 22.3 Hz– was hidden behind the walls of the room.

Seventy-nine volunteers participated in the study, all of whom had been told before spending time in the room that they might sense a presence, feel a tingling sensation, experience an anomalous smell, and so on. Each participant spent fifty minutes alone in the room, and was asked to record if, at what times, and in which specific locations, they experienced odd sensations. Some of them were subjected to EM pulses, others infrasound, some a combination of both, and others neither. "Most people reported at least some slightly odd sensation, such as a presence or feeling dizzy, and some reported terror, which we hadn't expected," explains French in an article published in *Scientific American*.

Although intriguing, the results of the experiment remain inconclusive. There appears to be little correlation between the "paranormal" sensations experienced by the participants and the EM field and infrasound activity, thus indicating that suggestion was to blame, that the participants experienced odd sensations because they expected to. Another contributing factor, notes French, is that the room, being quiet, dimly lit, and featureless, may have induced "a form of mild perceptual deprivation." Their inability to replicate Persinger's effect can perhaps be explained by the nature of their experimental set up, he adds. Persinger reminds us that for an EM field to have a noticeable effect on the brain, it must possess specific qualities – qualities that the EM fields used in French's study probably lacked.

In *Wrestling with Ghosts*, Sevilla explores the hypothesis that a connection exists between fluctuations in geomagnetic activity and the frequency of SP attacks. The human brain, he says, being an electrochemical device, is likely to be affected by geomagnetic influences. Sevilla has so far conducted two studies on the matter, the first of which concerned his own SP experiences. For a 23.5-month period, Sevilla kept a record of his SP episodes, while monitoring changes in the ambient geomagnetic field.

What he discovered seemed to confirm Persinger's findings: the "paranormal experiences" – in this case, his own SP episodes – occurred more frequently during periods of high geomagnetic fluctuation. The same was true of his lucid dreams. He eventually expanded his study, collecting 2, 972 observations from fifty subjects over a period of eight years, the results of which indicated that "the probability of a reported SP episode increased to 0.26 for either abrupt rising or declining global geomagnetic activity." Though his findings are intriguing, Sevilla's research is still at the stage where no hard conclusions can be drawn on the matter.

In a challenging paper entitled "The Most Frequent Criticisms and Questions Concerning the Tectonic Strain Hypothesis," Persinger gives an overview of the experimental work he has conducted to try and simulate the visitor/abduction experience. A common aspect of these experiences, he says, is that the victim feels the "sense of a presence." So do SP sufferers, as explained earlier, while so-called alien abduction encounters are popularly thought to be SP episodes. Although Persinger makes no direct reference to the SP phenomenon, he does mention that the sense of a presence can occur naturally during REM sleep, especially if one is in a state of emotional distress, or if one's nocturnal melatonin levels are running low. He writes: "It is the likely correlate of the sense of 'Muses' or 'Inspiration' reported by creative writers, musicians, poets and artists when they remain awake during the early morning hours..."

In an experimental procedure similar to that which Blackmore underwent, Persinger's subjects were exposed to weak, complex magnetic fields with the strength of about one microtesla (μT). The fields were first applied over the right hemisphere (temporoparietal lobes) for about fifteen minutes, then over the left hemisphere. Consequently, says Persinger, the subjects immediately experienced the "sense of a presence," previously mentioned. "Some subjects attribute it to a 'spirit,'" he says, "others attribute it to mystical sources. The affective polarity of the experience, i.e., negative or positive, will determine if the attribution is associated with a positive (god) or negative (demon) label." The outcome of these experiments can be better understood when one considers that the left and right hemispheres of the brain are two different "people" or "selves," says Persinger. It is thought, too, that awareness is focused in the left hemisphere – that we "live" in this part of the brain.

When the "other self" residing in the right hemisphere of our brain is stimulated, he says, allowing it to intrude into left hemispheric awareness, "the experience is that of an ego-alien 'presence.' Effectively this 'presence' is the other 'you.'" Because this "other self" "lives" in the emotional, creative right hemisphere and is "associated with hypervigilance and anxiety," according to Persinger, we're likely to perceive it as negative and frightening when we meet it face to face. (Hypervigilance is defined, by *Dorland's Medical Dictionary*, as "abnormally increased arousal, responsiveness to stimuli, and scanning of the environment for threats.") Persinger mentions, furthermore, that the "entity" is often identified as male by women, and as female by men, and that it usually appears on the left side of the body. These two details are of particular importance to our study.

One is immediately reminded of Gooch's "succubus" encounter, described in a previous chapter. In his opinion, of course, the female entity he made love to, although separate from himself, was in fact a manifestation of his unconscious mind, possessing "physical and even psychological attributes familiar to me." Perhaps Gooch is right. Maybe he did encounter his "other self" – though not necessarily his unconscious mind, but rather the "entity" living in the right hemisphere of his brain.

Is there a connection, I wonder, between the fact that Persinger's subjects sensed a presence on the left side of their body more often than their right, and the fact that the left side is of significance to schizophrenic patients and SP sufferers? The sinister voices heard by schizophrenic patients often appear to emanate from the left side of their body, while the same has been observed by SP sufferers, including myself. Furthermore, an SP sufferer is more likely to sense a presence on the left side of their body than their right. Are we dealing, then, with encounters between our left and right hemispheres, or with spirits? Or perhaps with a combination of both?

That Persinger has managed to stimulate the brain in such a way as to generate a "sense of presence" – a feeling frequently felt by SP suffers – does not in any way invalidate the "spirit hypothesis" put forward in this book. All it does is raise more questions. According to theoretical physicist Fred Alan Wolf in his book *The Dreaming Universe*, "there seems to be no doubt that imaginal-realm experiences are produced by electrical disturbances in the temporal lobe. These can be induced by anomalous electro-magnetic phenomena, such as those that accompany tectonic stress relief in the earth's crust and brain surgical procedures, and even under laboratory settings." But, he then asks, "what about you and me? *What about so-called normal people who, through seemingly no fault of their own, experience such phenomena when no added electrical stimulation is present?*" (my emphasis). What indeed?

To explore Persinger's theory in any great depth is beyond the scope of this book. There are many compelling arguments for and against it, and to explain them all would take up too much space. What cannot be denied, however, is that geomagnetic influences *may* play a role in the frequency of SP attacks, and that these experiences *do* involve an increase in temporal lobe activity – which is not to suggest that SP attacks are simply caused by abnormal brain function. All the evidence presented so far demonstrates that the SP phenomenon cannot be entirely explained by the mechanistic science of today. Even if you are unwilling to admit that SP experiences have a paranormal cause (in addition to a physiological cause), you would surely have to agree, at the very least, that the phenomenon remains a genuine mystery.

Although, in my view, it seems implausible that EM fields, caused by seismic activity and electrical appliances, for example, could influence one's brain in such a way as to make one think that one had had a complex and profound close encounter experience (or, for that matter, an SP attack), it cannot be denied that our bodies are EM systems, and that the EM radiation we are exposed to on a constant basis (both natural and man-made) profoundly affects us in a number of ways (both consciously and unconsciously). The nervous system, which is made up of billions of neurones, functions in an electro-chemical fashion and is susceptible to influence from EM fields outside the body of roughly the same frequency. It's been discovered, furthermore, that the body acts as a weak radio transmitter, and that even our muscles emit EM waves of various frequencies.

Especially damaging to our mental and physical health are those energies in the extremely low frequency range (ELF), both EM and acoustic (infrasound). ELF waves fall within the range of frequencies that are emitted by parts of the human body (from just above zero to about 100Hz) and can therefore disrupt the body's normal functioning. Because they have long wavelengths, ELF waves are extremely penetrating and have the remarkable ability to travel around the circumference of the earth, losing little energy in the process. Those who own a drum set (or are unfortunate enough to live next door to someone who does) would have noticed that the sound from the bass drum (which is low in frequency) can be heard much further away, and is much more difficult to block out, than the sound from one of the cymbals (which is high in frequency).

ELF fields surround almost all electrical appliances, including power lines, and are particularly strong near power transformers. A number of studies have indicated but not proven a link between regular exposure to strong ELF fields and a number of ill effects, including headaches, nervous tension, memory loss, epigastric pain, dizziness, depression, suicide, mood changes and irritability, restlessness, leukaemia, acute attacks of glaucoma, blood clotting, heart failures, and changes in oxygen metabolism. It is not uncommon for those who live in close proximity to mobile phone towers, ham radio towers, or power pylons, or for those who work in electrical-related professions, to develop some of the conditions just mentioned. Of course, people who believe in the harmful effects of EM pollution, and who claim that we're not being told the full story by our governments, are unfairly branded as kooks and conspiracy nuts, and tend not to be taken seriously.

In one German experiment, in which honeybees were confined to an area containing an EM field of 50Hz at 6,000 V/m (volts per meter), the bees became restless and aggressive, and even started attacking each other. Such fields are also known to slow down the heartbeats of rats. It should be borne in mind, however, that these same effects don't necessarily apply to humans.

In *The Cycles of Heaven*, written by Guy Lyon Playfair and Scott Hill, the authors mention the case of a California woman who "was made physically ill and almost driven mad" by her extreme hypersensitivity to EM waves, which she was actually able to hear. An electronics engineer investigated the case in-depth. The authors propose that many so-called lunatics who complain of hearing noises that others can't "may be just as sane as anybody else, only far more sensitive to their polluted sound or EM environment."

This brings us back to the subject of SP, for it seems to me that some of the sounds that SP sufferers hear can be explained as a result of one's body acting as a kind of "radio receiver" (which is not to suggest that one is *only* picking up radio waves). More specifically, it would appear that the SP state not only allows one to "tune in" to the spirit realm and thus hear the voices of discarnate entities, but also to various portions of the electromagnetic spectrum (perhaps the radio and microwave portions) that one cannot normally "pick up" – at least not while fully awake. Some of the electronic-type sounds reported by SP sufferers include buzzing and siren noises, and noises resembling "high pitched power tools."

There is a phenomenon called the microwave auditory effect (also known as the Frey effect), whereby clicking, buzzing, and chirping sounds induced by pulsed microwave frequencies can be heard directly outside, and also within, the head – even though others nearby may hear nothing at all. The effect was first reported during World War II by persons working in the vicinity of radar transponders and was later studied by the American neuroscientist Allan H. Frey. It occurs when microwaves heat, and therefore expand, parts of the human ear around the cochlea. It was later found to be possible, using signal modulation, to produce sounds or words in this fashion, presumably resembling the auditory hallucinations of SP sufferers and schizophrenic patients.

Technology of this kind has since been developed (and most likely perfected) by the U.S. military. As revealed in a deeply disturbing article published in the *Washington Post* in 2007, titled "Mind Games," the Air Force Research Laboratory (AFRL) has already patented a device that uses microwaves to transmit words inside a person's head. When the author of the article, Sharon Weinberger, filed a Freedom of Information Act request on this technology, the Air Force, she says, "released unclassified documents surrounding that 2002 patent – records that note that the patent was based on human experimentation in October 1994 at the Air Force lab, where scientists were able to transmit phrases into the heads of human subjects, albeit with marginal intelligibility." Whether or not research in this area is still taking place cannot be ascertained, as the AFRL refuses to disclose such information.

One wonders if the microwave auditory effect could account for some of the strange noises heard by SP sufferers, schizophrenic patients (like Mary, for example), and others whose minds appear to have the ability to access a greater portion of the EM spectrum than is normal.

In British UFO researcher Albert Budden's thought-provoking book, *UFOs: Psychic Close Encounters*, he puts forward the theory, called the Electro-Staging Hypothesis, that those who regularly have paranormal experiences, particularly close encounters, are EM hypersensitive (EH) and, while in the presence of EM radiation, have a tendency to experience visions of alien beings, apparitions, UFOs, and other strange phenomena. These "hallucinations," he believes, are produced by the unconscious mind in an attempt to integrate itself into consciousness. The unconscious, he says, "wants existence and expression in the conscious 'world,' rather like a genie that is cooped up within the confines of a bottle..." Budden's theory is not too dissimilar to what Gooch and other proponents of the "unconscious mind theory" believe, but with the added ingredient of EM radiation and its supposed effects on human consciousness.

Electromagnetic hypersensitivity, according to the World Health Organization (WHO), "is not a medical diagnosis, nor is it clear that it represents a single medical problem." The WHO has further stated that "there is no scientific basis to link ES [electrical sensitivity] symptoms to EMR [electromagnetic radiation] exposure." One medical professional who does take the condition seriously, however, is Dr. Sarah Mayhill, who is registered with the General Medical Council and practices privately in Wales, UK. In an article that appeared in the *Daily Mail* in 2007, titled "The Woman Who Needs a Veil of Protection from Modern Life," Mayhill is quoted as saying: "There is no doubt that electrical sensitivity is a real phenomenon – I have seen too many people affected by electro-magnetic radiation to think otherwise."

The condition is taken seriously by numerous other medical professionals all over the world who insist that it cannot possibly be psychosomatic. Those afflicted with EH often sufferer from a number of other allergies, including food and chemical allergies – as is commonly the case with alleged UFO abductees. The symptoms of EH sufferers include severe headaches and dizziness, high blood pressure, digestive and memory problems, hair loss, rashes – and, if Budden is correct, "epileptiform perceptions induced by field exposure."

Budden believes that EH sufferers are not only given to hallucinatory states, whereby they see alien beings, UFOs, and sometimes even ghosts, but may also become the focuses of poltergeist activity, producing PK phenomena that they believe to be caused by external, paranormal forces. Most abductees "have a history of psychic experiences," says Budden, "often reaching back to childhood and often including encounters with other entities and apparitions."

According to Budden's theory, EH occurs when people are exposed – usually over a long period of time – to unhealthy levels of EM radiation, causing irradiation; this sometimes happens in childhood. Afterwards, the presence of EM radiation induces an allergic reaction in these individuals, one symptom being that they emit their own personal EM fields, which can apparently cause electrical equipment in their presence to malfunction. The body, explains Budden, "re-radiates ambient fields, transforming them into a more coherent form...It is these 'beams' which interfere with aspects in the environment, often identified as poltergeist activity." Budden has found, time and time again, that many alleged abductees emit strong EM fields, as shown with the use of a field meter, and that they often live close to, or once lived close to, powerful sources of EM radiation.

In *Electric UFOs*, which expands on the information presented in *UFOs: Psychic Close Encounters*, Budden proposes that the "hallucinations" experienced by abductees are important messages from the unconscious mind, warning the individual that their health is threatened by harmful EM radiation. "Although the body apprehends these external and artificial fields as alien to its system," he explains, "the unconscious, in its symbolic communications to the conscious mind, will select imagery of aliens from its images banks, and will present it to the conscious mind as personalized alien forms."

This is, no doubt, an original and compelling theory, and may explain some cases of alien abduction, and perhaps some cases of SP. I wouldn't be surprised if it ends up being established that a significant number of SP sufferers are EM sensitive to some extent, for I myself occasionally experience headaches in the presence of florescent lights (which emit electric and radio frequency fields), and generally sleep better when the electrical equipment in my bedroom has been switched off.

Bearing in mind that my summary of Budden's work is much too brief, it's easy to see that certain aspects of his rather complex Electro-Staging Hypothesis are extremely difficult to accept, especially when we consider that a significant number of UFO sightings, poltergeist hauntings, and other paranormal events involve multiple witnesses – not all of whom could possibly be EH. Although, according to Budden, this can be explained by the supposed transmission of ambient fields from one mind to another, resulting in a group-hallucination effect, there is little evidence to suggest that this phenomenon is possible. Furthermore, and perhaps more importantly, one can't help but question whether it's actually possible for EH sufferers to experience vivid, life-like hallucinations as a result of EM exposure. Accepting, as I do, that the condition is real, where's the strong evidence to prove that hallucinations are one of its symptoms?

There is, I admit, a strong link between high EM activity and paranormal phenomena in general, and it seems to me that spirits, aliens, and other entities of this nature, being energetic beings, possess the ability to manipulate and harness various energies – not exclusively EM energy. In *Electric UFOs*, in a section on the Enfield poltergeist case, Budden attempts to convince the reader, somewhat feebly, that there were no spirits involved, that the paranormal activity that took place was due to Peggy Hodgson's house being located in an EM hot spot. I'm my view, however, in order to make at least some sense of this case, one must factor in the existence of one or more discarnate intelligences, *acting through, but independently*, of Janet.

During the Enfield case, Playfair and Grosse, using a magnetometer, discovered "that there was some link between poltergeist activity and anomalous behaviour of the surrounding magnetic field," as the needle of the device was sometimes observed to deflect at the exact same time that PK phenomenon occurred. Also, during the haunting the family's pet goldfish were found dead in the tank – something that the poltergeist claimed responsibility for. "I electrocuted the fish by accident," it declared. When Grosse asked what kind of energy was used, the poltergeist replied "'Spirits' energy." Asked if this energy was electrical in nature, the poltergeist said "No. Powerful."

I will attempt, in the remaining chapters of this book, to shed some light on the nature of "spirit energy," and how it relates to, but is distinct from, EM energy. One name given to this energy is "orgone," and it is said to have an antagonistic relationship to EM radiation. It would be a mistake to assume that, just because there is a link between high EM activity and paranormal phenomena, the former is responsible for the latter. It's much more likely, I think, that the former is a "side effect" of the latter, in the same way that the generation of heat is a side effect of incandescent lighting.

CHAPTER 15

Robert Monroe: Out-Of-Body Extraordinaire

Before he had his first out-of-body experience (OBE) in 1958, Robert Allan Monroe was an ordinary businessman, "living a reasonably normal life with a reasonably normal family," with little or no interest in anything to do with the "paranormal" or "occult." Born in 1915, his father was a college professor and his mother a medical doctor. After graduating from Ohio State University, where he studied engineering and journalism, Monroe spent some twenty years working as a creator and producer of radio and TV programs. He later formed a number of companies, the first of which was Robert Monroe Productions, which produced radio network shows. He also formed, and was president of, Jefferson Cable Corporation, the first cable-TV company to cover central Virginia.

Monroe was a highly intelligent, exceptionally driven individual and a successful businessman. In a personality profile featured at the end of his first book, *Journeys Out of the Body* (1971), psychiatrist Stuart Tremlow of the Topeka V.A. Hospital describes Monroe as "extremely independent," a "natural leader," and "highly creative." According to Tremlow, Monroe, like many others who experience OBEs, possessed certain identifiable personality attributes, such as "a tendency to feel socially isolated and different from others at quite an early age, often seeing the world itself as somewhat alien."

In *Journeys*, Monroe describes the circumstances of his life when his first OBE occurred. He had been living with his family in Virginia, in the peace and quiet of the country. And, he insists, the only "unorthodox activity" he had been doing at the time was listening to sleep learning tapes as part of an experiment to test their effectiveness. One Sunday afternoon, after listening to a sleep learning tape, then eating a light meal, Monroe began to suffer from a severe pain in his solar plexus, "a solid band of unyielding ache." He first suspected it was food poisoning, but everyone else in his family – all of whom had eaten the same meal – felt fine. The painkillers he took had no effect. The pain lasted till sometime around midnight, at which point he fell asleep "from pure exhaustion." When he woke up in the morning, he felt fine – the cramp had disappeared.

Several weeks later, while the family was away at church, Monroe lay down on the couch to take a short nap and was suddenly struck by what seemed like a beam or ray of warm light. It came down from the sky, he says, at about a thirty degree angle from the horizon. "Only this was daylight and no beam was visible, if there truly was one." The beam affected his body in such a way that he became paralyzed and began to "vibrate." "It was like pushing against invisible bonds." The paralysis soon faded, as did the vibration. Feeling a little shocked, he went outside for a walk. Over the following six weeks, Monroe experienced the same peculiar condition a total of nine times. It always happened in the same way. He would lie down to take a rest and find himself unable to move. Then the "vibrations" would begin. Every time it occurred, he would fight the condition, and it would soon pass.

As he doesn't mention the term "sleep paralysis" in any of his books, it's obvious that Monroe was ignorant of the condition – at least initially. This is not surprising, as *Journeys* was first published in 1971, when, as far as I can determine, little or nothing was known about SP. A doctor he visited, Richard Gordon, was apparently also unfamiliar with the condition. He subjected Monroe to a thorough examination but was unable to find anything wrong with him. Monroe was relieved to discover that he did not suffer from a brain tumor or epilepsy. Dr. Gordon told Monroe that he was probably stressed from overwork and recommended that he sleep more and lose weight.

Thinking that the condition "must be hallucinatory, a form of dreaming," and therefore entirely safe, Monroe decided to explore it a little more closely. When the condition next came on, he "stayed with it, trying to remain calm." Although frightened, he did not fight his way out of the experience, as he had done so many times before. Again, he felt a powerful sensation of vibration, "steady and unvarying in frequency. It felt much like an electric shock running through the entire body without the pain involved." The sensation was accompanied by a "roaring sound." Five minutes later, the condition faded away, and Monroe felt fine. From that point on, his attitude to the condition was no longer one of abject fear; he felt more curious than afraid.

The "vibrations" persisted, and on one occasion Monroe saw them "develop into a ring of sparks" about two feet in diameter. The "ring" surrounded his body, and remained visible when Monroe closed his eyes. It appeared to sweep back and forth across his body, from his head to his toes, completing one cycle every five seconds. "As the ring passed over each section of my body," he wrote, "I could feel the vibrations like a band cutting through that section." Whenever the ring passed over his head, Monroe felt the vibrations in his brain, and heard "a great roaring sound."

Before I continue with Monroe's story, I should point out that I, too, have seen a ring or band of energy surrounding my body. The experience occurred while I was deep in the SP state, with my eyes open. But, unlike Monroe's ring, mine did not move; it remained stationary. On this particular occasion, I did not experience any vibrations, nor did I hear any strange roaring or whistling sounds. In fact, very rarely are my SP attacks accompanied by these two phenomena. Other SP sufferers frequently experience "vibrations," a sensation that is usually accompanied by a loud noise. In Terrillon's and Marques-Bonham's aforementioned paper, published in the *Journal of Scientific Exploration*, the authors – both of them SP sufferers themselves – explore the connection between the SP phenomenon and various paranormal experiences, particularly OBEs. In a description given of a typical SP episode, the authors mention how one will often hear, at the beginning of the experience, "a buzzing/ringing/roaring/whistling/hissing/high-pitched screeching sound..."

Worried that he might be developing schizophrenia, Monroe confided in a psychologist friend by the name of Dr. Foster Bradshaw. He did not utter a word about his unusual experiences to his family. Bradshaw assured Monroe that mental illness was out of the question, suggesting that the phenomenon could be some form of harmless hallucination. Asked what he thought he should do about the situation, Bradshaw replied: "Well, there's nothing else you can do but look into it and see what it is."

Several months later, while lying in bed, waiting for the vibration to cease so that he could get to sleep, Monroe noticed that his arm was draped over the bed, and that his fingers were just touching the rug. Without giving it much thought, he tried moving his hand closer to the rug and was surprised to discover that his hand kept going, straight through the floor below it. Underneath the floorboards, he "felt" what appeared to be a triangular piece of wood, a bent nail and some sawdust. Extending his arm still further, Monroe felt water, which he splashed around with his fingers.

It took a moment for Monroe to realize that he was not dreaming. He was, he says, "wide awake" – or at least he felt that way. Looking out the window, he noticed that everything appeared normal. The landscape outside was bathed in moonlight. As the vibrations started to fade, Monroe began to grow worried that, if he didn't remove his arm in time, it would stay stuck in the floor. Perhaps, he thought to himself, the vibrations had made a temporary hole in the floor. He removed his arm with ease, the vibrations ended, and he sat up in bed. The following day, the idea occurred to him to cut a hole in the floor and see if what he had felt – the triangular piece of wood, etc. – actually existed, but he decided against it. After all, he thought, the experience was probably nothing more than a vivid hallucination. So why risk ruining the floor?

Four weeks later, the vibrations reappeared. As he lay in bed, not sure how to approach the situation, Monroe's thoughts turned to gliding – his hobby at the time. Moments later, he found himself lying against a wall – or what he thought was a wall. He suddenly realized that the "wall" was actually the ceiling, and that he was pressed up against it, "bouncing gently with any movement I made." Looking down, he saw a bed with two people lying in it, one of whom was his wife. But he was unable to recognize the man lying next to her. Monroe describes what happened next: "I looked more closely and the shock was intense. *I* was the someone on the bed!" Fearing that he'd died, or was in the process of dying, Monroe panicked, swooping down into his body, "and when I opened my eyes, I was looking at the room from the perspective of my bed."

More worried than ever, Monroe paid a second visit to Dr. Gordon, who ran further tests, including fluoroscopes, electrocardiograms, EEG, and numerous others. He even checked Monroe for indications of brain lesions. All the tests revealed a clean bill of health. Once again, Monroe confided in his good friend Dr. Bradshaw, explaining how he appeared to have floated out of his body. Dr. Bradshaw said he was familiar with the phenomenon, having heard about it in college, while studying Hinduism. "Some of the fellows who practice yoga and those eastern religions claim they can do it whenever they want to," he told Monroe. "You ought to try it." It struck Monroe as absurd that one would be able to leave one's body and fly around in spirit-form. Still, he decided to take Dr. Bradshaw's advice and approach the situation with an open-mind.

Some time later, while the vibrations were operating in full force, and while Monroe was feeling particularly courageous, he willed himself to float up out of the bed – and it actually worked. When he thought of going downward, he floated downward, and when he thought of moving to the side, his astral body moved accordingly. Only after many "test runs" of floating around the vicinity of his body then re-entering it was Monroe able to move around confidently in the OBE state. Learning to control his astral body required much practice, he discovered, just as learning how to drive a car requires much practice. Having verified, on countless occasions, that what he perceived while in the OBE state also existed in the "real world," Monroe was able to prove to himself that the experiences, instead of being dreams or hallucinations, were entirely real. Monroe presents numerous examples of this – of seeing something in the "OBE realm" or "astral realm" that is later proven to exist in the "real world" – in the first chapters of *Journeys*.

Curious by nature and scientifically minded, Monroe set about researching and exploring the OBE state, recording every one of his experiences. Unlike most people for whom OBEs are spontaneous once-in-a-lifetime events, Monroe had the rare ability to leave his body at will – relatively speaking, of course. Sometimes he was unable to relax sufficiently to achieve the state necessary for OBE traveling. But over time, with practice, leaving his physical body became increasingly easy, to the point where it required very little effort.

While in the OBE state, Monroe found it much easier to "home in" on people than to locate specific places. All he had to do was think of a particular person – usually someone with whom he had a strong emotional connection – and, almost instantaneously, he would appear in their presence. In one such "experiment," Monroe attempted to visit a friend of his – a businesswoman – whom he identifies as R.W. She was on vacation at the time, staying somewhere on the New Jersey Coast. In preparation to visit R.W., says Monroe, "I lay down in the bedroom...went into a relaxation pattern, felt the warmth (high order vibrations), then thought heavily of the desire to 'go' to R.W. There was the familiar sensation of movement through a light-blue blurred area, then I was in what seemed to be a kitchen. R.W. was seated in a chair to the right."

Two teenage girls accompanied R.W. All three women were drinking beverages and talking amongst each other. While R.W. was still engaged in conversation with the two girls, Monroe began to talk to her – not orally, but "superconsciously." Just to make sure that R.W. would remember the visit – which she mentally insisted she would – Monroe decided to pinch her just below the rib cage. Surprisingly, she actually reacted, jumping backwards and shouting "ow!" Monroe then returned to his physical body.

A few days later, when R.W. had returned to work, Monroe asked her what she had been doing on Saturday between three and four p.m. – when his "OBE visit" had taken place. She had been sitting in a beach cottage, she said, having a conversation with her niece and her niece's friend – both of them in their teens. She was having a drink, and the girls were having cokes. "Can you remember anything else?" asked Monroe; she said she couldn't. Feeling impatient, he then asked: "Do you remember the pinch?" R.W. looked astonished. She then lifted her sweater, exposing two bruises on the exact same spot where Monroe had pinched her. R.W. revealed that she had felt the pinch while talking to the two girls. It had taken her by complete surprise. "I turned around, but there was no one there," she told Monroe. "I never had any idea it was you!"

Interestingly, the incident seems to indicate that the astral body – or what Monroe prefers to call the "Second Body" – is able, under certain conditions, to affect physical matter. Also compelling is the fact that Monroe was able to talk to R.W. – or some part of her – without her having any conscious awareness of it. These "conversations," says Monroe, which appeared to be taking place between two superconscious minds (or, to put it another way, on a superconscious level of mind) occurred on frequent occasions. Monroe first suspected that he was imagining these communications. However, he says, "this theory received a setback when a number of such communications brought out data known only to the second party."

Assuming we each possess a superconscious mind, or higher self, it may very well be that we engage in conversations with spirits and OBE travelers all the time – while we're awake and while we're asleep – and that our conscious minds have no knowledge of these exchanges. Who knows, perhaps I'm chatting to a spirit as I write this very sentence. In a fascinating section on the "Occult Transmission of Thought," *The Spirits' Book* explains that "a spirit is not enclosed in his body as in a box, but radiates around it in every direction. *He can, therefore, hold conversations with other spirits even in the waking state, although he does so with more difficulty*" (my emphasis). The book goes on to explain that, on those rare occasions when two awake people appear to have the same thought at the same time, their spirits, being in sympathy, may have communicated with each other.

Examining his own astral body, Monroe discovered that there does indeed exist a "silver cord" linking it to the physical body, as declared by numerous occultists. Apparently, at death, this cord is severed, and you lose all connection with your physical body and consequently the "physical realm." The term "silver cord" is derived from Ecclesiastes 12:6-12:7 in the Old Testament, which states: "Or ever the silver cord be loosed, or the golden bowl be broken, or the pitcher be broken at the fountain, or the wheel broken at the cistern. Then shall the dust return to the earth as it was: and the spirit shall return unto God who gave it."

This "silver cord," according to Monroe, is connected to one's back, directly between the shoulder blades (of the astral body, not the physical body), and appears to be composed of hundred, possibly thousands, of "tendonlike strands, packed neatly together." This connection – which Monroe describes as more of a "cable" than a cord, due to its two-inch thickness – proved to be immensely flexible. According to one theory, this flexible quality allows the silver cord to stretch across apparently infinite distances, becoming longer and longer the further away you travel from your physical body. Monroe's writings neither confirm nor deny this theory. (Is there, I wonder, such a thing as distance in the astral realm, anyway? It would seem that there isn't, that in the astral realm distance does not exist as we conceive of it.)

Monroe observed that the sense of touch in the astral body is similar to that in the physical body. He says, furthermore, that the astral body can touch physical objects, and that you can also feel your physical body; although this is only possible when you are located in the physical world – what Monroe calls "Locale I." In addition to Locale I, he says, there are two other "realms" or "dimensions" that one can travel within, each one separated by a different frequency. He refers to them as "Locale II" and "Locale III."

In *Journeys*, Monroe describes a series of unusual OBEs that appear to shed some light on what occurs to the astral body during the SP state. On several occasions, the moment he had left his physical body, Monroe felt and heard what appeared to be someone lying next to him, "a body, warm and alive, pressed against my back." He could tell the "presence" was male and could even feel whiskers on its neck. Monroe first concluded that the "entity" was an "adult male, panting with passion, thoroughly sexually deviated." Perturbed, he returned to his body as quickly as possible.

When next in the OBE state, Monroe again felt the "pervert" on his back, breathing heavily in his ear. But this time he didn't react in fear, deciding instead to investigate the situation. Reaching back, Monroe put his hand on the "man's" face; it felt exactly like his own. When he held his breath, the "man" behind him stopped panting. He did it again, and the same thing happened. His own breathing, and that of the "body" behind him, was exactly synchronized. He then realized: "The warm body clinging to my back was me!" But, thought Monroe, although both bodies were his own – the one in front and the one behind – which one was his physical body and which one was his astral body? He soon concluded "that the one in back – the one I could hear and feel – was the physical 'I,' and the 'I' in front was the mental or real 'I.'" In other words, the "man" clinging to his back was his own physical body.

What had happened, in a sense, is that Monroe's consciousness had become split between his physical body and his astral body, creating the impression that the former did not belong to him, that it was somebody else. Had he been properly out of his body – as opposed to "just out of the physical," as he puts it – this strange phenomenon would presumably not have occurred. Considering that the SP state involves, in some cases, a partial dislocation of the astral body from the physical body, could it be possible, I wonder, that when an SP sufferer feels or senses a body lying next to them (as has happened to me on a number of occasions), they are actually feeling or sensing their own physical body?

In a short section in *Wrestling with Ghosts*, entitled "Out of Phase Dual Awareness," Lucy Gillis explores the fascinating theory that some SP attacks could be one's attempt to re-enter one's physical body following an OBE journey. Such journeys, she suggests, may occur every time we drop off to sleep, yet we are unable to remember them – a concept we're already familiar with. There is a difference, she says, between the way time operates in the dreaming state, and the way time operates in the waking state. Sometimes, for instance, one will be dreaming for what seems like hours, when only a few minutes have transpired in the "real world."

"What if," asks Gillis, "besides this time distortion, there can sometimes also be a time lag? What if our bodies experience sensations that may have had their origin only seconds before, but the cause of those sensations (the dream) is forgotten, like some out-of-phase dual awareness?" To help explain her theory, Gillis cites an OBE experience reported by Jorge Conesa, when, after leaving his physical body, he had difficulty trying to re-enter it. "So I approached my sleeping body and began chewing on and biting my own toes so I would wake up."

Gillis asks: "What if, in the out of body state, we encounter difficulties getting back into the physical bodies? (Or, if not 'out of body' we encounter difficulties in waking up and we hallucinate a dream version of our waking body.) What if we do like Jorge and attempt to get back in (or wake up) by alerting the physical body, trying to stir it into wakefulness? Could some of the sensations felt during sleep paralysis be an 'echo' of this activity when the mind switches from dreaming consciousness to waking?"

Gillis's theory could perhaps apply to Monroe's "pervert on the back" experience. His experience seems to indicate – just as Gillis's theory suggests – that some SP sensations can be attributed to an odd effect whereby one's awareness has become split between one's physical body and one's astral body, thereby producing the feeling that one is in the presence of an alien entity, when in actual fact this "entity" is a part of oneself. As Gillis so aptly asks, "Could we ourselves be the 'demon' sitting on our own chests…?" Assuming this theory is correct, it would mean that the SP state is a kind of "consciousness glitch," in that one's astral body has not properly separated from the physical body. The similarity between this theory and Persinger's "right hemispheric intrusion" theory will not have escaped the reader's attention. Both of them are suggesting much the same thing – that SP experiences are a kind of "confrontation" between two separate parts of oneself.

Described in *Journeys* are several OBEs in which people living in Locale I – what Monroe sometimes calls "the here-now" – were able to perceive Monroe's astral body. One such experience occurred in 1962, when Monroe decided to pay R.W. another astral visit. He entered the living room of her apartment and found her sitting in a chair, wide-awake. She looked directly at him and became frightened. The experience ended moments later, when Monroe woke up; he had been sleeping on his arm, and the lack of circulation was giving him "pins-and-needles." The following day, R.W. told Monroe of an unusual experience she had had the night before – an experience that, because she knew of his OBE activities, she felt related to him. She had been sitting in the living room, reading the paper, when "something made me look up, and there, on the other side of the room, was something waving and hanging in the air." It looked, she told him, "like a filmy piece of grey chiffon."

Because, concludes Monroe, the astral body is visible under certain conditions, "it must either reflect or radiate light in the known spectrum, or at the least a harmonic in this area." In a chapter dedicated to "visual manifestations," *The Mediums' Book* explains that the spirits of the dead, as well as those of the living (i.e. OBE travelers), are able to render their "semi-material envelopes" – i.e. their perispirits – visible when required. The ethereal perispirit is normally invisible, states *The Mediums' Book*, but is able to undergo "modifications that render it perceptible to the sight, whether by a sort of condensation, or by a change in the molecular disposition: it then appears to us under a vaporous form."

The perispirit is said to have properties similar to that of a fluid and is sometimes referred to as a "fluidic envelope." But, even though it's "fluid-like" in nature, it does not literally condense when it becomes visible; rather, the word is used metaphorically to give some idea of the means by which this process takes place. Water, of course, has three states of being – solid, liquid, and gas. When water vapor – which exists as a colorless gas – undergoes a process of condensation, forming into tiny liquid water droplets in the air, fog and cloud is formed. Further condensation results in the formation of dew – a liquid. The perispirit undergoes a similar kind of process when it transforms from a visible state to an invisible state, and vice versa.

According to Monroe, the astral body is not entirely immaterial, for it does possess weight, and is also subject to gravitational attraction but to a far lesser extent than the physical body. Perhaps, he suggests, the astral body's ability to pass through solid objects can be explained in terms of mass – it possesses so little density, and therefore hardly any mass, "as to be able to sift through the space between the molecular material structure."

As confirmed by many psychics, as well as by those who have witnessed "spirit phenomena," such as the kind that can occur in haunted locations, the perispirit or astral body can change shape, and, while in motion, will often take the form of a sphere or orb. Apparently, the shape of the astral body is entirely up to its "wearer." (I use the word "wearer" because the astral body could be considered a piece of clothing – a kind of garment for one's soul.)

In *Far Journeys*, the sequel to *Journeys*, Monroe compares the constitution of the astral body to that of gelatin, describing it as "much like gelatin that has been removed from a mould." The astral body possesses a "memory" of the physical body, he says, and therefore looks almost identical. But this memory can fade over time as well as "distance," meaning that the longer you are away from your physical body and the further "away" you travel, the more this "memory" will wane, causing you to appear less and less humanoid in form. "If left to its own devices," says Monroe, "you may become a ball, a teardrop, a small cloud, or just a 'blob.'" Given this information, perhaps it's not surprising that when people see spirits "going about their business" – such as I have following SP attacks – they're commonly spherical in form.

In *Far Journeys*, Monroe explains how he discovered that we possess not one astral body but two. It all started when, as a fairly experienced OBE traveler, he began to notice that it required more effort than usual to re-enter his physical body. He had always experienced some resistance during the process – as is typical – but in this case the resistance had become too much. During one particularly difficult attempt to re-enter his body, Monroe, in his own words, "pulled back slightly, stopped trying, and examined the problem." It looked as though his physical body had split into two.

This "other body," he observed, was positioned adjacent to his physical body, about four inches away, and was almost identical in appearance, only less dense. Monroe attempted to merge with it and was successful. He writes: "It seemed as if I were partially interspersed with the physical, yet not quite in phase. The condition had a familiarity that took me all the way back to the vibration I first encountered and the physical paralysis that went with it. The sensation was near-identical..." Once "inside" this "second astral body," discovered Monroe, little effort was required to move into his physical body. He had solved the problem of resistance.

Having learned conclusively that he did indeed possess a "second astral body," Monroe, when returning to the physical, would always re-enter it first and then slip into his physical body. This eventually became an automatic process. Monroe discovered that the "second astral body" "hovered" near the physical, while the furthest away it could move was about ten to fifteen feet. The astral body, on the other hand, once released from the "second astral body," was free to move anywhere; it was not restricted by distance.

Monroe says that your form, while in the OBE state, needn't necessarily have substance, and that if you slips out of your "second astral body" immediately after separating from your physical body, you can become "clear undiluted energy," a kind of "energy essence." This observation of Monroe's – that "proper" OBE travel requires an exit first from your physical body then a "second astral body" – may be of significance to our understanding of the SP state. It would seem to suggest that many SP episodes, maybe most, do not involve a full entry into your astral body but instead takes place while you are occupying your "second astral body." Monroe said that while occupying the latter body, you feel as though you are "partially interspersed with the physical, yet not quite in phase," and that the condition involves a state of paralysis accompanied by vibrations. This is an almost perfect description of the SP state.

When, on one occasion, Monroe entered the OBE state intending to visit a friend, he instead found himself floating above a busy street. He immediately recognized his whereabouts – the main street of the town where his friend lived. But, he asked himself, why hadn't he arrived at his friend's house – or, more correctly, in his friend's presence? Following the sidewalk, he arrived at a gas station on the corner where he noticed a white car parked out the front, situated near two open doors, its rear wheels removed. Monroe couldn't understand why he'd arrived at this particular destination.

Disappointed, he returned to his physical body.

Feeling impulsive, he jumped in his car and drove the five miles to the town where his friend lived (he does not give a name). He wanted to inspect the location he had visited while in an OBE state. When he arrived at the gas station, he saw a white car parked out the front, situated near two open doors. He immediately recognized the vehicle as the one he had seen during his OBE journey. Positioned above him were electricity pylons – a source of powerful EM radiation – leading Monroe to speculate that perhaps electric fields attract the second body. He later found out that his friend had been walking down the street at the exact same moment of his OBE journey, and that, as far as they could determine, Monroe had been floating directly above him, following him along.

Occultists have long known that EM radiation – more specifically magnetism – can affect the aura, of which the astral and etheric bodies are a part. The etheric body, according to Constable in *The Cosmic Pulse*, is composed of orgone energy, which can be influenced by, and has an antagonistic relationship with, EM radiation. As for the astral body, Constable says it's "of emotional substance" and therefore "not accessible to physical detection." On this point Monroe would disagree. Proof that the astral body is not entirely immaterial, and that it's subject to influence by certain natural forces, such as electricity and gravity, was revealed in a fascinating experiment in which Monroe was placed in a faraday cage and asked to enter an OBE state.

The purpose of a Faraday cage is to block out all EM radiation, thereby shielding whatever or whoever is placed inside. They are sometimes used as environments in which to test electronic components or systems that are sensitive to EM interference. The Faraday cage in which Monroe was placed had a charge of 50kv D.C. Having left his body, Monroe says he "seemed to be entangled in a large bag made of flexible wire. The bag gave when I pushed against it, but I couldn't go through it." The electric field produced by the cage seemed to be repelling Monroe's astral body. Realizing that he couldn't penetrate the cage, Monroe returned to his body. "Maybe," he suggests, "this could be the basis for a 'ghost catcher!'"

Not all of Monroe's OBEs took place in Locale I. Most of them, in fact, took place in Locale II. There are several reasons for this, the most significant one being that Locale I proved difficult to move around in. Moving in Locale I is comparable to swimming in cloudy water, he says, as it is not the natural environment of the astral body, just as the ocean is not the natural environment of man. In Locale I, you are unable to see with very much clarity, while most of what you perceive registers in shades of black and white. Monroe discovered that finding your way around Locale I is something of a challenge. Whenever he attempted to go to a specific place – such as the house of a friend – he would often get lost.

Monroe describes Locale II as a "non-material environment with laws of motion and matter only remotely related to the physical world. It is an immensity whose bounds are unknown…and has depth and dimension incomprehensible to the finite, conscious mind. In this vastness lie all of the aspects we attribute to heaven and hell." This "dimension," says Monroe, "seems to interpenetrate our physical world," and possibly exists on a higher vibratory level. To explain its "location," he uses an analogy we're already familiar with – that of various wave frequencies in the electromagnetic spectrum. Monroe describes Locale II as being made up of various rings or layers, which surround the physical world like the many layers of an onion, each one higher in vibratory frequency to the one preceding it. Therefore, the "further away" one travels from the physical plane, the higher the frequency becomes.

In Locale II, says Monroe, "thought is the wellspring of existence…As you think, so you are." This can sometimes cause problems, he adds, particularly for those who have difficulty controlling their emotions. Being in Locale II forces you to realize that you are far more emotionally repressed than you had previously thought, and that most of your actions are dominated by your emotions, particularly by various fears. Not until Monroe had learned to harness his "uncontrollable emotional patterns" was he able to think and act rationally in the OBE state. It could be said that the OBE condition is a person's true condition, in the sense that you are "naked" and unable to conceal your true nature. Your soul remains totally exposed.

According to Monroe in *Journeys*, Locale II is populated by non-physical beings of both human and non-human origin, while the majority of those who inhabit the areas "nearest" to the physical world are "insane or near-insane, emotionally driven beings." These entities sound a lot like hungry ghosts. A large number of these beings, he says, appear to have become "trapped" after death and are incapable of "moving on." The rest of them, as far as he could determine, are the spirits of the living, who, having fallen asleep, are drifting around Locale II in a state of unconsciousness, almost like zombies. They are "alive but sleeping." According to *The Spirits' Book*, many people in this condition – asleep and in the OBE state – "give free reign to their passions, or remain inactive." Only those who have attained a certain degree of spiritual accomplishment do anything particularly purposeful or useful with their time in the astral realm.

In *Far Journeys*, Monroe explains a little more about the nature of the "hungry ghost realm" – which, he repeats, is an area that lies closest to the physical realm and which is "just slightly out of phase with physical matter." Some of the inhabitants of this ring, he explains, once lived on Earth but after death were unable to accept the fact that they were no longer physical. "Thus they kept trying to be physical, to do and be what they had been, to continue physical one way or another. Bewildered, some of them spent all of their activity in attempting to communicate with friends and loved ones still in bodies or with anyone else who might come along, all to no avail. Others were held attracted to physical sites…"

As soon as you leave your body, says Monroe, you pass within the vicinity of this "hungry ghost realm," an area where you are likely to meet all sorts of unpleasant characters, many of whom have not yet learnt to control their sex drive and desperately crave sexual satisfaction. In *Far journeys*, Monroe describes encountering a huge "sex pile" – a seething mass of males and females "so focused and intent on seeking sexual satisfaction they were unaware of any other existence…" Considering that this realm lies closest to the physical realm and is "just slightly out of phase with physical matter," coupled with the fact that SP involves a partial dislocation of the astral body from the physical body and could easily be described as a condition in which one is "just slightly out of phase with physical matter," perhaps it's little wonder that SP sufferers are usually "visited" by spirits who come across as troubled "emotionally driven beings."

As far as spirits who were attracted to physical sites – ghosts, that is – Monroe encountered many during his OBE trips. Once, while living in a rented house positioned over a small river, Monroe went to bed and was in the process "of lifting out of the physical" when he saw a white form, shaped like a woman, move into the room. His wife lay asleep beside him. The white form approached the side of the bed, and Monroe was able to see her clearly. She looked middle-aged and had straight dark hair. Her body was transparent. Monroe sat up in bed – "non-physically, I'm sure" – and reached out to touch her. "What are you going to do about the painting?" she asked him. Not sure what to say, Monroe said he'd take care of it and told her not to worry. The woman smiled, clasping his hand between both of her own. "The hands felt real, normally warm and alive." The woman walked out the door and was never seen again.

A few days later, speaking to a neighbor named Dr. Kahn, Monroe learned that the previous owner of the house – a Mrs. W – had died about a year ago in the very same bedroom that he and his wife were sleeping in. The house had been her pride and joy, the neighbor told Monroe; she had decorated it with many beautiful paintings. Dr. Kahn showed Monroe a photograph of the woman standing among a group of people. Without knowing which particular face belonged to Mrs. W – there were fifty to sixty people altogether – Monroe was able to identify her. Dr. Kahn looked surprised at first, then assumed that Monroe had come across a photograph of Mrs. W in the house somewhere. Monroe nodded in agreement; he did not mention the fact that he'd seen the woman's ghost!

"Tell me," asked Monroe, "did she have any unusual mannerisms?"

"Why, yes," replied Dr. Kahn, "whenever she was happy or grateful, she took your hand in both of yours, palm to palm, and gave a little squeeze."

In *Journeys*, Monroe describes the time he was attacked by a group of hectoring spirits while staying the night at his brother's house. His four-year-old niece was asleep in the next room, with their beds positioned against a common wall. As soon as he lay down in bed and began to relax, Monroe felt the vibrations come on. He decided to leave his body for a moment, "just to test being in this condition away from home." As soon as he did so, Monroe noticed the presence of three malevolent beings in the room. They began to approach him; Monroe hovered close to his physical body, not sure what to do. Like a group of schoolyard bullies, the entities began to shove him around, pushing him this way and that. "They were having a good time at it," he says. "I wasn't sure I could get back into the physical quickly enough before they pulled me away."

Thinking he was doomed, that there was nothing he could do to evade the situation, Monroe began to pray to God, pleading for his help. He also prayed to Jesus Christ and several Catholic saints. His tormentors found this hilarious and began to shove him around more forcefully than before. "Listen to him pray to his gods," one of the entities chuckled. Angry, Monroe began to fight back, pushing the entities away from him. Soon he had enough room to dive into his physical body. The moment he "woke up," Monroe heard the sound of his niece crying in the room adjacent to his. She had, it turned out, had a particularly bad night terror and continued crying for a very long time, unable to regain full consciousness. "Was my niece's trancelike nightmare a coincidence?" asks Monroe. In a later chapter of the book, Monroe explains how someone operating in the OBE state can affect another human being mentally, as demonstrated, for example, by the aforementioned "pinching incident." Most of these effects, he says, "may show in nothing more than sleep disturbances." Presumably this would include SP.

Intriguingly, in a chapter in *Journeys*, Monroe describes a series of encounters with beings whose nature resemble those I have termed elementals. He calls them "intelligent animals." Believe you me, the surprise I experienced when I read this chapter was immense. Monroe's observations dovetail my own perfectly. Monroe's first encounter with an intelligent animal occurred in 1960. He had just separated from his body and was hovering about eight inches above it, when he saw *out of the corner of his eye and to his left*, a small humanoid creature about the size of a ten year old boy, three feet tall with thin limbs, little pubic hair, and undeveloped genitals. The entity was clearly male.

What happened next is best explained in Monroe's own words: "Calmly, as if it were a daily occurrence – like a boy swinging onto his favorite horse – he swung a leg over my back and climbed onto me. I could feel his legs around my waist, his small body pressed against my back. I was so completely surprised that it didn't occur to me to be afraid…I waited rigidly, and by rolling my eyes to the right, I could see his right leg hanging over my body, less than two feet away. It looked like a perfectly normal ten-year-old boy's leg…I was still hovering just out of the physical, and cautiously wondering who and what this was. 'He' seemed completely unaware that I knew of his presence, or if he was, he didn't care."

Not wanting to confront the entity, Monroe quickly returned to his physical body. He mentions that it did not "have the feeling of human intelligence," but "*seemed more animal, or somewhere in between*" (my emphasis). Monroe was perturbed and insulted by the fact that the entity acted so casually and with such indifference. "He seemed confident that he would not be detected, perhaps through long association with humans to whom he was invisible."

About a week later, during the onset of an OBE in which he experienced vibrations throughout his body, Monroe felt something climb onto his back – it was the "little fellow" from his previous OBE. The entity grabbed onto his back and wouldn't let go. While the vibrations continued, Monroe, using one of his non-physical hands, reached down his side and grabbed hold of one of the entity's legs. "The consistency felt much like flesh, normally body-warm, *and somewhat rubbery*; it seemed to stretch" (my emphasis). As he attempted to pull the entity off of him, the more it stretched and the more it struggled to climb back on. Unable to dislodge the entity, Monroe began to panic, re-entering his physical body (although, to be accurate, he hadn't completely left his body).

When he next attempted to leave his body, Monroe noticed that the entity was still clinging to him. And this time there was not one but two of them. Monroe floated over to the center of the room, all the while struggling to yank the entities off his body. He began to scream for help. Holding one entity in each hand, Monroe took a closer look at them. Each began to change shape, transforming "into a good facsimile of one of my two daughters." Monroe then adds a joke in brackets – "The psychiatrists will have a good time with this one!" – and continues: "I seemed to know immediately that this was a deliberate camouflage on their parts to create emotional confusion in me and call upon my love for my daughters to prevent my doing anything more to them." The reader will recognize the similarity between this experience and Gooch's "succubus encounter." In both cases, the entity (or entities) encountered took on a sexually or emotionally appealing form, in order to make their "victim" think or behave in a particular way.

The moment Monroe recognized that they were "playing with his mind," the entities changed back into their true form. He attempted to scare them away by thinking about fire (and presumably burning them), but this had little effect. "I got the impression that they were both amused, as if there was nothing I could do to harm them." Just when Monroe was about to lose hope, a serious-looking man entered the room and gently removed the entities from his body. "As he held them," says Monroe, "they seemed to relax and go limp, limbs and necks drooping." Monroe speculates that the entities may have been thought-forms, which he unintentionally created through certain habitual thought patterns.

Featured in Constable's *The Cosmic Pulse* are several black and white photographs of what have been labeled "atmospheric fish." The photographs, which were taken with infrared film, appear to show a "school" of these entities sweeping past the camera. In what may be a coincidence – or perhaps something more – Monroe describes, in *Journeys*, a couple of encounters he had with "astral parasitic sucker fish." Between eight and ten inches long, they attached themselves to various parts of Monroe's astral body, causing quite a nuisance. Luckily, they weren't vicious and didn't appear to cause any harm. As soon as Monroe had managed to remove one of the creatures, it would come back or another one would take its place. To escape them, Monroe decided to return to his body. On another occasion, Monroe found himself surrounded by them. As before, they attached themselves to his astral body. But this time he didn't flee. He waited patiently, and after a moment the fish detached themselves and moved away.

One time Monroe was attacked by an entity "about four feet long, like a large dog" that "seemed pure animal." He fought it in the darkness of his hotel room "for what seemed an eternity." Only after the battle was over, and Monroe had thrown the creature out the window, did he realize he was not in his physical body. During another encounter with a demon-like entity, Monroe tried in desperation to defend himself, while his attacker applied pressure to his nerve centers, causing excruciating pain. The fight went on for what seemed like hours. Just when he thought he couldn't go on any longer, when he thought his very soul was going to be annihilated, Monroe managed to slip back into the safety of his physical body. Fortunately, the entity did not return.

Originally published in 1985, Monroe's second book, *Far Journeys*, is a highly unusual work. The second half of the book is written in an almost novelistic fashion. In it, Monroe visits a number of "dimensions" or "realities," including Earth in the future, explores his past-lives, and talks and interacts with a multitude of non-physical entities, some of them more evolved than humans. Understandably, some sections of the book are a little difficult to swallow, but for the most part it's surprisingly convincing. However, it's the first-half of the book that concerns us here because in it Monroe explores some fascinating research on the OBE state, which just happens to reveal a lot about the truly paranormal nature of the SP phenomenon and how these experiences involve contact with spirits. Monroe's findings show that the SP state – or what he refers to as the "borderland sleep state" – is not only conducive to OBEs and lucid dreaming but to mediumship as well.

Monroe established The Monroe Institute (TMI) – "a non-profit educational and research organization dedicated to the exploration of human consciousness" – in the late-1970s (although its origin dates back to the mid-1950s, when Monroe and his colleagues began conducting research into audio sleep learning technology). Following the publication of *Journeys* – which generated a great deal of public interest in OBEs – Monroe, with the intention of helping others explore the OBE state, initiated research into methods of altering consciousness with the use of sound. Monroe and his colleagues discovered that various sound patterns can affect the brain in such a way as to induce altered states – one of which they labeled Focus 10, a condition in which the mind is awake and the body is asleep, and OBEs come naturally.

This technology became known as Hemi-Sync (short for Hemispheric Synchronization), and is still popular today. With the use of a pair of headphones, separate sound pulses are sent to each ear, and, explains Monroe, "the halves of the brain must act in unison to 'hear' a third signal, which is the difference between the two signals in each ear." This third sound is called a binaural beat. If, for example, one hears a sound measuring 100 in one's left ear, and a signal of 125 in one's right, the whole brain – meaning both hemispheres – will "generate" a signal of 25. Depending on the signal that the whole brain "generates," different states of consciousness result. A signal of 25, for instance, may induce a state of deep relaxation, while a signal of 22 might assist with memory retention. Whatever the signal may be, both hemispheres of the brain are made to work in unison; they become synchronized, in other words, allowing people to harness their whole-brain potential. Or so it is claimed, anyway. The technology remains somewhat controversial.

The Focus 10 state is similar, if not identical, to the SP state. In Focus 10, the person appears, physiologically speaking, as though he or she is in a light or deep sleep, says Monroe. The state is characterized by EEG activity showing "a mix of waves ordinarily associated with sleep, light and deep, and overlaying beta signals (wakefulness)." As part of the Gateway Program (or Voyage), which still runs to this day, attracting people from all over the world, participants lie down in enclosed bunks or CHEC units (Controlled Holistic Environmental Chambers) and are made to wear headphones, allowing them to listen to consciousness altering hemi-sync sound. The units feature microphones so that the person inside can communicate with a monitor. Electrodes attached to the body read the participant's physiological activity – brain wave, etc. During a typical session, the monitor guides the participant into various altered states – the first one being Focus 10, whereby, according to Monroe, "the mind is slightly out-of-phase with normal physical wakefulness."

Beginning in Focus 10 (mind wake, body asleep), the participant is guided into a more expanded state of awareness called Focus 12, whereby, "all physical-data input is shut off and consciousness can reach out and begin to perceive in ways other than through the five senses." In this state, colors, shapes and pictures are likely to appear in your mind. Journeying further, the participant reaches Focus 15, a "state of no time," followed by

Focus 21, "the edge of time-space where it's possible to contact other energy systems." To journey beyond Focus 21 is to leave one's physical body and enter the astral realm.

At one point, says Monroe, he and his colleagues sent their OBE participants out beyond the solar system with the intention of finding intelligent life. At first they were unsuccessful, and "it seemed to us a sterile universe," he says. But that all changed in 1974, when an affirmation was developed for the program, which each participant was encouraged to say at the beginning of their session. Part of it went as follows: "…I deeply desire the help and cooperation, the assistance, the understanding of those individuals whose wisdom, development, and experience are equal to or greater than my own." The introduction of this affirmation had the effect of attracting the attention of a large number of intelligent non-human beings, all of them eager to communicate. In fact, says Monroe, these entities made their presence known almost every time a participant had an OBE, or entered an advanced Focus 12 state. Some of the participants communicated with these entities telepathically, and even formed close friendships with them, sometimes interacting with them on a regular basis.

One participant described meeting a "green man" – not just once, but on multiple occasions. The entity, who dressed in a green robe, told the participant that he was his overseer, "somewhat responsible for my growth and development." Another participant – an electronics engineer – described, over the microphone in his CHEC unit, an encounter with an entity who told him that the Earth is his "territory," and that there are other entities like him who have the same role. As to what this role might be, the participant received the impression that they "are made available to us to help us maximize or get through our earth experience."

Four or five of these "spiritual guides" formed a close relationship with one of the female participants, an office worker. In a session transcript included in *Far Journeys*, the woman describes how the entities "helped to lift my energy body out," after which she felt "real light and really, really good." The beings then asked her if she wanted to try an experiment, to see if one of them – the spokesman of the group – would be able to use her body as "a transmitting set between dimensions" (that is, talk through her using her vocal cords). She agreed. A moment later, the woman began to speak in a totally different voice. She – or rather, the entity speaking through her – spent ten minutes lecturing the monitor about "other dimensions" and "other levels of consciousness," concluding his speech with the words, "It is a privilege. Thank you, dear friends."

What the entity imparted was identical in content to so much other channeled material. Monroe found some of it quite compelling. He and his colleagues hoped that their non-physical friends would provide them with the answers to some important spiritual questions. And so the channeling continued. Whenever the woman was in her CHEC unit and had entered the appropriate altered state, she would be met by her spirit friends who would position themselves around her, two on each side, then lift her out of her body. Most of these sessions took place on a Wednesday at five o'clock. But one week the woman had to cancel, and someone else – a female psychologist – took her place instead. Skeptical of Monroe's research, the psychologist had decided to visit to see what all the excitement was about. Monroe suggested that she take part in one of the sessions and experience the phenomenon for herself.

Five minutes after the woman had entered the booth, Monroe heard her voice on the intercom speaker. "There is someone else in the booth with me," she told him. Monroe couldn't believe his ears. "As a matter of fact," she added, "there are four of them. I can perceive them very clearly. There are two at my feet and two at my head." Monroe asked her what the beings were up to. She replied: "They are trying to lift me out of my body." According to the woman, the entities spent a moment arguing amongst each other; then went away. They had, it seems, mistaken her for the other woman, who normally occupied the booth at five o'clock on a Wednesday!

Monroe and his colleagues recorded hundreds of hours of channeled material, most of it of a philosophic nature. Some of it took the form of suggestions and advice concerning the personal well being of the participants. When contact was first initiated between an entity and a participant, says Monroe, the entity would usually appear in the form of a hooded figure, its face hidden in shadow. Then, as the participant became more comfortable with the entity, it would discard its robe. And although the participant would not be able to see its face, they would still be able to sense its radiation and therefore its presence.

Monroe notes that whenever one of entities borrowed a participant's vocal cords and spoke through them, their vocabulary would be limited to that of the participant. This, of course, is a well-established fact of mediumship. *The Mediums' Book* goes a step further on this point, stating that, if a medium is not in sympathy with the spirit (or spirits) from whom he's receiving and transmitting a communication, "he may alter their replies and assimilate them to his own ideas and propensities." But, the book continues, "he does not influence the spirits themselves: he is only an inexact interpreter."

Significantly, Monroe mentions that these apparently highly evolved entities had "total access" to the memory of the person through whom they communicated – i.e. the medium. And, he adds, not only were they able to manipulate the medium's vocal cords but their breathing apparatus and body temperature as well. Many of the participants described how, when interacting with these entities, the entities made use of a kind of "soul technology," which enabled them, among other things, "to remove the energy essence of a human from his physical body without disrupting his biological systems." Once the person's body had been "vacated," the communicating entity would then be able to "enter it," and thus control it to some extent.

One particular "device," which was a part of this technology, seemed to involve the use of counter-revolving discs and looked, according to one participant, "like two big eyes." The exact purpose of the device could not be ascertained. The participant described being placed on one of the discs, which began to spin around. "They are spinning me around on this disc, and shooting a light beam on me…There is light over all my body. I think the light is coming from the other disc which is over me. It is as if I am between two energy discs." Participants described, time and time again (supposedly hundreds of times), encountering this "soul technology" and the apparently benevolent beings responsible for its operation. These bizarre experiences share something in common with alien abduction episodes, but without the fear and trauma. There is much mention of bright lights and odd sensations, such as being touched by warm, friendly hands. "I can feel a lot of energy between their touch and my energy body," reported one participant. "It feels good…it is a tingle…they are going to work on little spots on my feet. My toes. My big toe. Their fingers are now just working on my big toe."

When the entities spoke through the participants – which was not always an easy process, involving, in some cases, much fine tuning of vocal cords – what they had to say was nothing particularly special – at least not by today's standards. These days, of course, there is an abundance of channeled material available, and everything that's going to be said by our discarnate "teachers" in the next dimensions has probably already been said. Although he hasn't been recognized as such, Monroe was clearly a channeling pioneer, as his (unintentional) investigation into the phenomenon began at a time when it had not yet come into its own. Monroe, of course, began receiving channeled information (through his Gateway participants) in 1974 – just two years after the publication of Jane Robert's *Seth Speaks*, which is credited with initiating the channeling craze. The popularity of the phenomenon peaked in the 1980s and is now beginning to make a comeback.

During one channeling session, a transcript of which is included in *Far Journeys*, one entity, talking through a social worker, raved on and on about different levels of consciousness and how as people evolve spiritually their level of consciousness supposedly increases. Plants, according to the entity, "are on a vibrational rate on the levels one through seven," while animals "exist on the levels eight through fourteen." Humans, moreover, being a different "form of consciousness" to plants and animals, occupy much higher levels on the consciousness scale – from fifteen to twenty-one, to be exact. Once a person has reached level twenty-eight, "the bridge is crossed, and from that point on for a consciousness to evolve higher, it would not again assume human form of any kind..." It had already "crossed the bridge," said the entity, and would never incarnate again as a human being.

To discuss these "spiritual teachings" further would be really quite pointless, because not only is the information dull but, as Monroe points out, it poses more questions than it answers. "We thought our 'new' associates would provide answers," he writes. "But for every answer, at least fifty new questions arise..." As a result, Monroe and his colleagues wisely moved on to other areas of research.

What's important, however, is not the fact that these entities may have been lower astral entities, but the very fact that mediumship took place. Remember that whenever this phenomenon occurred, Monroe's participants were either in an OBE state, which shares much in common with the SP state, or in an advanced Focus 12 state. What we have here is a definite link between the SP phenomenon and the realm of the paranormal – more specifically, contact and communication with spirits. I should mention, too, that the kinds of experiences Monroe's participants underwent while interacting with these beings, such as being touched, for example, or hearing spirit voices, are similar in nature to SP experiences, including some of my own.

It should be clear by now that SP episodes occur on an astral level, involving, in some cases, a partial dislocation of the astral body from the physical body, including a strange effect where the person's consciousness becomes divided between the two, creating a sense of dual-awareness. Now, it would appear that the astral body departs from the physical body regularly during REM sleep, perhaps entering Monroe's "Locale II." However – and this is important – the astral body may not always travel far from the physical body but may simply hover nearby, like a helium-filled balloon attached to a string.

Monroe explores the same theory in *Journeys*. In some cases, he says, the distance of separation may only be a fraction of an inch, while in others it may be limitless. According to New Age author Robert Bruce – who has written numerous books on the topic of astral projection, one of the most popular being *Astral Dynamics* – your astral body "projects out" every time you sleep. "Normally," he says, "this hovers just above the physical body, mimicking its sleeping position. In effect, the projected double is out of body every night."

Assuming that the astral body leaves the physical body every time we fall asleep, and that the SP state involves little more than being awake and aware during REM sleep, it would not be unreasonable to state that the only real difference between an SP sufferer and a non-SP sufferer is that the former has some awareness of these astral experiences, these interactions with non-physical beings, and is able to remember them in the morning, while the latter has none. The same principle applies to dreams. Every one of us dreams, but the only people who think they dream frequently are those with good "dream recollection." Support for this theory can be found in an experience I described earlier, in which I woke up hearing a voice that said, "Why do you want to leave this place?" As I explained, the question sounded so casual, as though the being who asked it were an acquaintance of mine, and we were having a relaxed conversation. Could it be possible that we were, in fact, having a conversation – this spirit and I – and my slipping into a state of awareness is what turned the experience into an SP attack?

CHAPTER 16

WHITLEY STRIEBER AND THE VISITORS

A large part of the available UFO literature is closely linked with mysticism and the metaphysical. It deals with subjects like mental telepathy, automatic writing and invisible entities as well as phenomena like poltergeist (ghost) manifestation and 'possession.' Many of the UFO reports now being published in the popular press recount alleged incidents that are strikingly similar to demonic possession and psychic phenomena. – Lynn E. Catoe, *UFOs and Related Subjects: An Annotated Bibliography*

Anyone who knows anything about the subject of UFOs and alien abduction would have heard of Whitley Strieber, the successful horror novelist, who in 1987 published a book called *Communion*, which still stands as one of the most terrifying and powerful accounts of alien abduction ever written. Now a host of the online radio program Dreamland, which covers the latest news in paranormal phenomena, Strieber hasn't stopped writing and talking about the mysterious non-human beings he calls the "visitors."

Strieber came up with the term "visitor" to replace "alien" because he does not necessarily believe that aliens, in the true sense of the word, are behind the close encounter phenomenon, preferring instead to leave the question of their origin open until further evidence comes to light. Plus, he considers the word "alien" to have a negative connotation. The word "visitor," on the other hand, could not be more neutral; he chose it for this very reason.

The grays, says Strieber, are just one of the many different types of non-human being, or visitor, with whom he has been in close contact. "These people were not androids or robots. They were complex, richly alive beings who were obviously incredibly and totally different from us," he says. The grays feature commonly in accounts of alien abduction and are believed to be behind much of the UFO phenomenon witnessed in our skies.

Strieber was already a successful author before he decided to risk his reputation by publishing *Communion*. His previous books, of which there are many, deal with issues like nuclear war and environmental catastrophe. Along with childhood friend James Kunetka, Strieber wrote the 1984 *New*

York Times bestselling novel *Warday*, which concerns the subject of nuclear holocaust. He also wrote a number of highly acclaimed horror novels, such as *The Hunger* and *The Wolfen*, both of which were adapted into films.

When *Communion* was first published, it quickly shot to number one on the *New York Times*, non-fiction bestseller list. It then went on to become an international bestseller. Although Strieber allegedly received six figures from publishing company William Morrow (now an imprint of HarperCollins), it seems unlikely that *Communion* was a hoax and that he wrote it for the money, as some critics have claimed. In a 1987 interview for the *San Francisco Examiner*, Strieber said: "I didn't need to write it. I could have written another novel...Why would I hold myself up to the ridicule that a book like *Communion* brings? I felt that I had to write this book."

Following the publication of *Communion*, Strieber went on to write four additional books about his intimate contact experiences, each one (with the exception of *Confirmation*) far more "spiritual," and a little more "out there," than the last. First came *Transformation*, then *Breakthrough*, then *The Secret School* and, lastly, *Confirmation*. Along the way, Strieber lost some of his readership – those who wanted to read about his bloodcurdling abduction experiences, rather than the spiritual significance of the contact phenomenon.

Referring to these books in an interview, *Communion* and *Transformation* in particular, Strieber described them as "texts about the articulation of certain questions." What is important about these books, he said, "is the way they lead you to thinking about questions about the nature of perception and what exactly the physical world is." Considering that Strieber was a student of the Gurdjieff Foundation for more than fifteen years, it is perhaps not surprising that his work revolves around such matters. "Gradually I branched out from the readings from Gurdjieff himself and the people around him to much deeper studies," he says. Speaking about his spiritual orientation in a recent interview, Strieber remarked that he was brought up a Roman Catholic and has always considered himself one.

By far the most ambiguous of Strieber's books about the visitors is *The Secret School*. Strieber claims to have been contacted by the visitors from a very early age, and it is in this book that he explores some of those childhood memories, many of which, he says, remained repressed for a very long time. As a child growing up in San Antonio, Texas, in the 1940s and 1950s, Strieber says he lived a kind of double life in which he and numerous other "child abductees" belonged to a "secret school" run by the visitors. While a member of this school, Strieber was taught nine important lessons, presented in three triads. The first lesson involved an apparently non-physical journey to Mars, where Strieber caught a glimpse of the so called "Face" many decades before the first satellite photographs of the Cydonia region were taken in 1976 by the Viking Orbiter.

The Secret School is primarily concerned with the subject of time-travel and how this relates to prophecy. "The nine lessons," writes Strieber, "involved the manipulation of time, because learning how to use time as a tool is the key to reaching higher consciousness..." Unbelievable as it sounds, Strieber claims to have physically journeyed through time on a number of occasions. According to him, the ninth lesson of the secret school involved such an experience, whereby, in the summer of 1954, at age nine, he found himself suddenly transported into the future.

During the experience, Strieber saw a flat-screen TV, obviously unlike any kind of TV available in 1954. The TV was tuned to a news channel, and on the screen he saw a number of scenes that have "remained in my mind all of my life – not exactly as a conscious memory, but rather as a reservoir of visual images that I have come to draw on in my work." Some of the scenes were of catastrophic events that appear to have since come true, such as the Great Malibu Fire of 1993.

In his book *The Uninvited*, British UFO expert Nick Pope gives a humorous description of the time he met Strieber in London in 1996. Pope mentions that Strieber "seemed *so* casual about the most bizarre experiences. Here was a man, I suspected, who would describe these [visitor] encounters in the same sentence as an account of a trip to the shops, and might well use the same tone of voice." Slightly critical though these words sound, Pope says he did not find Strieber to be "a crank and an eccentric," as some believe him to be.

Assuming Strieber is telling the truth about his experiences, it would not be a stretch to classify him as a kind of shaman, an intermediary between this world and the world of the gods – the gods being the visitors. In an interview with Sean Casteel, Strieber made a comment that seems to support this view: "You know, Sean, I wonder who the hell I am. I wonder who I am...There are many things that have happened that I've never even put into books. Just incredible. *It's like I live with my two feet in two different worlds.* [my emphasis] And they're both equally real." In the introduction to his book *The Key*, Strieber makes a similar statement: "I have had the incredible privilege of living between the worlds, in the sense that I have actually spent a substantial amount of time in my life with people who were not physical in the way that we know the physical."

If Strieber is indeed a shaman of sorts, it might help explain an alleged incident that occurred in the pre-dawn hours of June 6, 1998, in which Strieber met an apparently human man who claimed to "belong to many worlds." Strieber says he was awoken by the man knocking on his hotel room door. As soon as he opened the door, the man burst into the room. They then proceeded to have a "remarkable" conversation about spiritual matters. Strieber took notes. He describes the man, whom he calls the "Master of the Key," as someone "in possession of the most incredible knowledge that I've ever encountered in my life about the meaning of mankind. Where we came from, where we're going, what's happening to us and why."

The Key, which Strieber self-published in 2001, is a transcript of this discussion, though it is not an exact transcript because Strieber says his notes did not cover the entire conversation word for word. Some of it he committed to memory. Interestingly, he says the notes "had a strange quality to them, as if each word was capable of causing a whole spring to flow in my mind," and that they "unlocked something in my mind." This comment seems to suggest that Strieber is able to produce automatic writing, and that he may be a channel for the visitors.

Having discovered "that there's a LOT down inside me that comes slipping out when I am in the trance-like state that writing fiction involves," and in an attempt to get "my inner self to tell me what I really know about the grays, and keep hidden," Strieber wrote a novel about these beings and the U.S. Government's clandestine involvement in the UFO phenomenon. Entitled *The Grays* (2006), sections of the book are written from the perspective of these entities in a very convincing manner, indicating that Strieber has a profound understanding of the way their minds operate.

Although the alien abduction "program" has essentially come to an end, with fewer and fewer people having physical encounters with the visitors, according to Strieber, mental contact with these beings continues; this, in fact, is the primary form of communication that's currently taking place. "I experienced this myself, and continue to experience it," explained Strieber in a 2003 journal entry. Once again, the possibility that Strieber is a channel for the visitors seems very likely indeed.

As those who have read *Communion* will know, Strieber had his first conscious meeting with the visitors on December 26, 1985, while staying with his wife and young son in their secluded cabin in upstate New York.

They also owned an apartment in New York City. But it was at the cabin that they spent most of their time, as Strieber preferred to work in the peace and quiet of the country. On December 26, a cold and snowy day, the Strieber's spent hours outside, cross-country skiing and breaking-in their son's new sled. After a meal of Christmas leftovers, the family retired to bed. For reasons he didn't know at the time, Strieber had become obsessed with security, and every night after arming the burglar alarm, he would secretly make "a tour of the house, peering in closets and even looking under the guest-room bed for hidden intruders." This night was no exception.

Later that night, Strieber was suddenly awoken by a "peculiar whooshing, swirling noise" coming from the downstairs living room. It sounded, he says, "as if a large number of people were moving rapidly through the room." Strieber sat up in bed, glancing at the burglar-alarm panel nearby; the system was still armed, he noticed. He then observed a figure, about three-and-a-half feet tall, standing behind the bedroom doors. Most of its body was concealed. It moved closer to the bed, allowing Strieber to make out some of its features. The being had "two dark holes for eyes and a black down-turning line of a mouth that later became an O." It seemed to be wearing an armor-like breastplate, and looked almost like a robot. Strieber notes that he was full awake at the time, with a clear mind, and could not have been in a hypnopompic state. He continued to sit up in bed, too stunned to do anything, all the while thinking that the figure must be a vivid hallucination.

Without warning, the figure rushed into the room, and Strieber somehow lost consciousness. A moment later, he found himself naked and paralyzed, being carried through the woods. He knew, at this stage, that he was neither dreaming nor hallucinating, that what he was undergoing was real. Following another brief period of unconsciousness, Strieber found himself in "a messy, round room," encircled by alien beings. His surroundings seemed cramped and stuffy, and the air was noticeably dry. He tried to move, but found his body still paralyzed. He felt like an animal caught in a trap. "The fear was so powerful that it seemed to make my personality completely evaporate."

Strieber saw small beings rushing around him at great speed – a sight he found "disturbing." Two beings were standing nearby, one on his left and one on his right. One of them, he could sense, was a female. Strieber recalls seeing many different species of alien being, some of them typical-looking grays, others with wide faces and short, stocky physiques, dressed in dark-blue coveralls. One of the beings – "a tiny, squat person" – showed him a strange object, "an extremely shiny, hair-thin needle." Strieber received the impression that the object was to be inserted into his brain, and this caused him to panic. He remembers telling the beings, "You'll ruin a beautiful mind." He then heard a voice with a "subtle electronic tone to it," ask "What can we do to help you stop screaming?"

Next, they performed an operation on his skull involving the needle he had been shown. The procedure happened very quickly, and all Strieber experienced was "a bang and a flash." A moment later, "an enormous and extremely ugly object, gray and scaly, with a sort of network of wires on the end" was inserted into Strieber's rectum, causing him to feel as though he were being raped. From what he could gather, the purpose of the device was to obtain a sample of fecal matter. Strieber recalls that an incision was then made on his forehead – an apparently painless operation. The next thing he knew, it was morning.

Following the incident, Strieber's personality "deteriorated dramatically," and he became moody, "hypersensitive," and "easily confused." He had difficulty sleeping, felt as though he were being watched, and was unable to concentrate for any length of time. Also, an infection appeared on his right forefinger, and he experienced a pain behind his right ear. Examining the area, his wife noticed the presence of a tiny scab. "My skull ached and the skin was sensitive," he says. Strieber felt that something extremely disturbing had happened to him but was unable to remember exactly what it was.

Gradually, though, he began to remember fragments of the incident, as well as fragments of other inexplicable experiences. He recalled, for instance, an odd incident that occurred on the night of October 4, 1985, when two friends – a couple named Jacques and Annie – were staying over at the cabin. During that night, Strieber was awoken "by a distinct blue light being cast on the living room-ceiling." He thought the house was on fire. But before he was able to act, he inexplicably fell into a deep sleep.

Later that night, he woke up again, "this time by a loud report, as if a firecracker had popped in my face." He heard his son and his wife cry out. The house was surrounded by a glow, and Strieber thought the "fire" had spread to the roof. Within seconds the glow disappeared, and everyone went back to sleep. The following morning, Strieber and the others said very little about the incident, almost as if nothing had happened. About a week later, however, a "very clear and dramatic" memory popped into Strieber's mind "of a huge crystal standing on end above the house, a glorious thing hundreds of feet tall, glowing with unearthly blue light."

Later, when he asked his son about the night of October 4, and if he'd had any unusual dreams, his son mentioned seeing, in a "dream," "a bunch of little doctors." He described the "dream" as the "strangest" he'd ever had, "because it was just like it was real." When he questioned Jacques and Annie about the strange events of that night, Jacques said he'd been woken up at 4:30 a.m. by a light shining in the bedroom. It was so bright he initially thought it was daylight and that he must have overslept. Annie reported hearing "the scurry of feet" across Strieber and Anne's bedroom floor, a noise she attributed to their cats. But this was not possible, as they had left their cats at their apartment that weekend.

Strieber heard of the respected UFO abduction researcher Budd Hopkins, author of *Missing Time* (1981), and decided to contact him. Something, he knew, was terribly wrong, and he needed to find answers. Perhaps, he thought, he was losing his mind. Hopkins listened to his story with interest and understanding. Through Hopkins, Strieber was put in touch with a therapist and hypnotist by the name of Dr. Donald Klein of the New York State Psychiatric Institute. Dr. Klein, who was open-minded about the alien abduction phenomenon, assessed Strieber as perfectly sane, as did numerous other highly qualified mental health professionals. As is often (but not always) the case with close encounter victims, Strieber could recall very little of his traumatic abduction episodes. In order to move forward and to come to terms with whatever was happening to him, Strieber needed to explore these "buried memories" – which is exactly what he did with Dr. Klein, starting on March 1, 1985.

The first hypnosis session concerned the events of October 4, 1985, when Strieber thought the cabin was on fire. Under hypnosis, he recalled going to bed rather early. Jacques and Annie, who slept in the guest-room downstairs, also had an early night. Strieber was woken up in the middle of the night by a light flying past the window. He then saw a dark figure, about three feet tall, hiding in the shadows. So frightening was the memory of seeing this being – "glaring at me from right beside my bed in the dead of night" – that he emerged spontaneously from hypnosis. "All I can say is that I relived fear so raw, profound, and large that I would not have thought it possible that such an emotion could exist," explains Strieber in *Communion*. Fully awake but unable to move, Strieber saw the being, a typical-looking gray, whom he could sense was female, approach him suddenly, holding a silver, wand-like object. Next, he says, the being touched him on the head with the "wand," "sticking in into my mind."

Being struck by the wand presumably had the effect of causing the loud noise – the "explosion" – that Strieber's wife and child reported hearing. As revealed under hypnosis, it also had the effect of producing images in Strieber's mind, one of which was of the Earth blowing up, "a whole big blast, and there's a dark fire in the middle of it and there's white smoke all around it." (This image, by the way, is something that many abductees have reported seeing during close encounter episodes.) Speaking telepathically, Strieber heard the being say: "That's your home. That's your home. You know why this will happen." Strieber interpreted the image as depicting a possible future scenario – one that could occur if environmental problems continued to be neglected. He also saw an image of his son sitting in a park, his eyes entirely black. He associated the image with death, and felt that his son might die if he didn't help him. Strieber speculates that the incident with the wand may have been a form of psychological testing.

On March 5, 1986, Strieber was hypnotized again to uncover more buried abduction memories, this time concerning the events of December 26, 1985, when he was subjected to a medical-like examination. As Strieber could recall, one of the beings he encountered was female. Under hypnosis, he mentioned recognizing this entity, "whose gaze seemed capable of entering me deeply." It was revealed, furthermore, that the device Strieber thought was used to obtain a sample of fecal matter had a different purpose altogether and was, in fact, an electroejaculator. As the name implies, an electroejaculator, which consists of a rectal probe and power control system, is a device used in animal husbandry to stimulate erection and ejaculation quickly, so as to obtain sperm samples from studs, for example. It would appear that Strieber was "anally probed" for a logical reason after all.

In March of 1986, Strieber's wife, Anne, was placed under hypnosis to see if she could shed some additional light on what was happening to her husband, and to see if she, too, had had any contact with the visitors. In the first session, which focused on the events of October 4, Anne recalled that the night had been a restless one, and that Strieber was absent from bed for a long period of time. She stated, in fact, that Strieber is frequently missing from bed at night. "He goes sometimes at night," she said. "He goes and works. Or he just goes." According to Strieber, however, he never works in the middle of the night. (In cases of alien abduction that involve a couple, in which one member is an abductee and the other is not – and this of course applies to Strieber and his wife – the non-abductee will usually be fast asleep and cannot be awoken while the abduction is in progress.)

Later in the session she stated that, on the night of October 4 (although it could have been the night of December 26, as the two dates became confused in her mind), Strieber left because "he was supposed to go." Later, she said: "They came for Whitley." She never stated exactly who "they" were. Using some kind of "mind control" technique, the visitors, it seems, had prevented Anne from revealing – or knowing – too much about Strieber's involvement and interactions with these beings. "I've often felt," she said under hypnosis, "that there are things going on with Whitley that I wasn't supposed to know. I'm supposed to kind of help him afterwards to deal with it. That's my role." Anne further stated that "they" came to Strieber "because of his head. He has a very unique head."

Further proof that the visitors had (and presumably still have) absolute control of not only Strieber's, but also Anne's, mind, can be found in a fascinating anecdote recounted in *Communion* – an anecdote that explains how the book got its title. According to Strieber, one night in April 1985, while contemplating whether or not he should call the book *Body Terror*, Anne, in a mediumistic fashion, said the following words in her sleep: "The book must not frighten people. You should call it *Communion*, because that's what it's about." Strieber notes that she spoke in a "strange basso profundo" voice, which he recognized straight away as belonging to the visitors. Strieber claims, like many abductees, that the visitors are able to speak both aurally and telepathically. When he heard one of the visitors during his December 26 encounter say, "What can we do to help you stop screaming?" the voice was definitely aural, he says. "It had a subtle electronic tone to it," he adds, "the accents flat and startlingly Midwestern."

Recounted in *Communion* is another anecdote of this nature, this time involving a different type of "medium." From 1970 to 1977, says Strieber, he and his wife lived in Manhattan, in a two-room flat on the top floor of an old building. One evening in April 1977, while sitting in the living room together, they suddenly heard a voice speaking through the stereo. It was, claims Strieber, "entirely clear" and "not like the sort of garbled messages sometimes picked up from a passing taxi's radio or a ham operator." The stereo had neither a microphone nor a cassette deck and had just finished playing a record when the voice came through. Astonishingly, Strieber and Anne were able to converse with the voice. "I do not remember the conversation," says Strieber, "except the last words: 'I know something else about you.'" It's possible, of course, for stereos to pick up interference from ham radios and police radios and such, but this doesn't explain how Strieber and his wife were able to speak back to the voice; the technology would simply not have allowed it.

The UFO literature abounds with such cases. In his book, *The Haunted Planet*, for instance, John A. Keel relates a mysterious incident that resembles Strieber's experience. Apparently, in January 1954, people throughout the Midwestern U.S. heard a strange voice, which spoke in a dull monotone, issuing from turned-off radios. "I wish no one to be afraid," it stated, "although I speak from space. But if you do not stop preparations for war, you will be destroyed." This same message, according to Keel, was apparently also picked up by equipment at the London airport, also in January of 1954. Schizophrenics, as we know, commonly hear voices from turned-off radios.

Like many abductees, Strieber's life is filled with inexplicable occurrences, not all of which are directly related to the alien abduction phenomenon. Another good example – one of many – can be found in *Communion*. Referred to by Strieber and his wife as the incident of the "white thing," it occurred sometime in 1981 or 1982. (An exact date is not given.) At that time, Strieber and his wife were living in an apartment in Greenwich Village, Manhattan. One night Anne woke up screaming, claiming that something had poked her in the stomach. She managed to catch a glimpse of the culprit, which she described to Strieber as "translucent white and about three feet tall." The incident was dismissed as a nightmare. (The similarity of this experience to an SP attack cannot be ignored.)

The following evening, while lying in bed, reading, Strieber was struck on the arm by the very same entity that Anne had encountered. He chased the entity – a "small, pale shape" – into the hall, but it disappeared. When he awoke in the morning, Strieber noticed a bruise on his arm, located on the exact same spot where the entity had struck him. Several days later, the white thing made another appearance, this time scaring Strieber's son who woke up "screaming the house down." In Strieber's words: "He said that 'a little white thing' had come up to his bed 'and poked me and poked me.'" Strieber's son had not been told about the previous two encounters with the white thing and thus knew nothing about the entity. To top it all off, while Strieber and Anne were away at a wedding reception one evening, the baby sitter who was looking after their son also saw the white thing, describing it as a "child in a white sheet." While cooking dinner in the kitchen, she noticed it peering at her from the fire escape. "We suddenly realized there was something weird about the white thing," says Strieber.

The 1989 *Communion* film was directed by Philipe Mora, a friend of Strieber's, whose work includes such B-grade movies as *Pterodactyl Woman over Los Angeles*. Like Annie and Jacques, and apparently many others, Mora witnessed some very strange phenomena while staying overnight at the Strieber cabin. On the evening of his visit in the summer of 1987, Strieber and Mora saw odd lights moving in the sky above the cabin, some of which may have been satellites and meteors. But at least one of the lights behaved in a very peculiar fashion, and neither Strieber nor Mora were able to explain what it was.

Mora describes what happened next: "Then we all went to bed...I was relaxing. I had the experience of lights blasting through the bedroom window, lights blasting under the crack under the door of the bedroom – I tried to turn the light on in my room, and I couldn't turn it on and I was pushed back into the bed. All the while I was consciously saying to myself, 'This is a hell of a nightmare.' Then I remember being outside the guest room door, in the kitchen area, and the whole cabin lit up – every opening, every exterior opening, the whole thing was lit up with moving lights."

In *Communion*, Strieber explores a large number of possibilities as to what the visitors might be, even suggesting that they may be us from the future or complex hallucinations caused by EM radiation. He draws some interesting comparisons between the visitors and the various types of entities that appear in fairy lore, such as goblins, gnomes, elves, pixies, leprechauns, and other ethereal beings. Like the ufologist and scientist Jacques Vallee, Strieber believes that our perception of the visitors may depend on our own cultural background. "They are an objective reality that is almost always perceived in a highly subjective manner," he explains.

Due partly to its highly mystical nature and to the fact that it has an almost occult flavor, Strieber's second book on the visitors, *Transformation*, wasn't as widely-received as *Communion*. Which is not to say, of course, that *Communion* isn't mystical also. In *Transformation*, Strieber begins to learn from the visitors; he sets off, one might say, on a spiritual journey of sorts – one that continues right through his other works on the visitors. He begins to recognize, moreover, that the visitors are neither angels nor demons, but, like us, possess both a positive and a negative side.

Of all the close encounter experiences detailed in *Transformation*, the one that occurred on December 23, 1986, is among the most fascinating. Strieber and his family had arrived at the cabin, where they intended to spend Christmas. That night, Strieber witnessed an unusual light in the sky, "too bright and close to be a plane." He then went to bed, waking up at 3:30 a.m. to go to the bathroom. When he returned to bed, Strieber began to feel "a tingling, pulsing energy running up and down my body." He also sensed a presence in the room and felt as though he were being watched – a feeling "so strong that it fascinated me. I would characterize it as a sensation of having another consciousness inside my mind. It was like being watched from the inside." (Was Strieber perhaps in the SP state?) After a brief period of unconsciousness, Strieber awoke to the sensation of someone slapping him on the shoulder. There, standing beside the bed, was a female visitor, an entity whom he felt he recognized. Strieber notes that she moved in a sudden, jerky fashion, much like an insect. (Interestingly, many abductees compare the visitors to insects.)

Wanting to take a picture of the entity, Strieber tried reaching for his camera, which he'd left beside his bed, fully loaded with film, for just such an opportunity. But, as he was about to grab it, his hand moved away of its own accord. The entity, he felt, was controlling his mind. Strieber found himself standing up, and with the entity positioned behind him, he began walking towards the bedroom door. Whenever he stopped and tried to resist, he would start floating along the ground, the entity pushing him from behind. "I could feel myself moving," explains Strieber. "I was passing through a normal and completely real version of my house."

This time the cats had been brought to the cabin, and one of them, Sadie, was crouched on the back of the couch, as if she were about to jump off at any moment. Strieber grabbed her as he floated past, cradling her in his arms. His reason for doing so, he says, was to determine whether or not his perceptions were being distorted; they appeared not to be. The visitor, Strieber, and his cat, all moved out the front door, at which point Strieber could no longer see normally; before him was a "glittering blackness." He could still feel the cat in his arms, though, whose companionship he found comforting. A moment later, he was standing in a room, with no idea how he got there. Before him was a desk and a bookcase stacked with books, including Thomas Wolfe's *You Can't Go Home Again*, which, curiously, was "pulled partway out of the shelf, as if to draw attention to it."

As well as his cat and the female visitor, Strieber was accompanied by three other beings, two men and one woman, none of whom were entirely human in appearance. The first man, who, as Strieber humorously puts it, "looked like something from another world wearing the clothes of the forties," had "a very, very long face" and "round, black eyes," and was seated behind the desk. Strieber's description of this individual makes him sound like a cross between a visitor and a human. (Such "hybrid" beings are commonly reported by abductees.) The second man, standing on Strieber's left, was tall and blonde with a flat face. His expression, says Strieber, "was gentle and touching and full of pity." The woman had fair skin and brown hair, and looked quite young.

Strieber sat down, and the man behind the desk began to speak. In normal English, he asked Strieber why he brought the cat along. "I'm reality testing," he replied. He describes their reaction to this comment: "They looked at each other as if I were completely crazy." For some reason, says Strieber, he felt compelled to speak the absolute truth, as though "a sort of mental pressure [were] being exerted on me." Strieber continues: "'I've made the cats a part of my life,' I heard myself saying. It felt like this was a deep, deep truth. 'They have to be taken when we're taken. They have to participate in the life of the family. It's their right.'"

Strieber was then told that the cat needed to be put to sleep temporarily. And so, using an instrument that looked "like two triangular pieces of brass with rounded edges," the cat was given what seemed like an injection. It instantly went to sleep. Strieber was asked, again by the man behind the desk, if there was anything they – the visitors – could do to assist him, to which he replied, "You could help me fear you less."

"We will try, but it will be very hard," Strieber was told. The device that had rendered the cat "as still as death" was also applied to Strieber's neck, leaving behind a red mark on his skin, which he discovered the following morning. During the next phase of this absolutely baffling encounter, Strieber was "pushed" back to the cabin. Still accompanied by the entity and under her control, Strieber entered his son's room and gently placed the "limp" cat on his bed. As soon as they reached his own bedroom, Strieber felt perfectly normal and fully awake. Turning around, he caught a glimpse of the female visitor standing in the doorway. Feeling unbelievably tired (a feeling induced by the visitor), Strieber collapsed on his bed, falling asleep instantly.

The following morning, Strieber found the cat where he had left it. It was still fast asleep, curled up in a ball beside his son's head. When it finally woke up, sometime after supper, it drank an "enormous amount" of water and was suffering from a stiff thigh – this being the spot where it had been "tranquilized" by the brass object. For a long time afterwards it wasn't quite the same, says Strieber, and "would sit staring for hours." One friend commented that it seemed "shocked." Eventually, however, the cat "returned to her usual, open curious self."

In the experience just described, a skeptic would probably declare that

Strieber underwent an SP attack – hence the sensed presence and tingling sensation – then fell asleep, entering an extremely vivid lucid dream featuring aliens and levitation. As for the cat's odd condition – this, they'd say, is certainly no proof that it was taken to an "alien world" and given an injection. Where, they'd ask, is the hard, physical proof? And how convenient, they'd add, that when Strieber went to photograph the visitor it caused his hand to move away.

When we consider that alien abduction experiences take place in the dead of night, usually just after the victim has been sleeping, and that the victim's body is often paralyzed for the duration of the encounter, we can see how easy it is for skeptical-minded individuals to explain these experiences away as frightening SP episodes – especially if the more "farfetched" details are ignored. Although it has to be admitted that there are some very obvious similarities between the two phenomena, it cannot be denied that there are many unmistakable differences too. Clearly we're dealing with two separate, but closely related, phenomena.

But dismissing Strieber's October 4 encounter as an SP attack is utterly ridiculous. That Jacques saw an extremely bright light shining into the bedroom; that Annie heard the "scurry of feet" across Strieber and Anne's bedroom floor; that Strieber's son "dreamed" of the "little doctors"; that Strieber recounted, under hypnosis, an extremely vivid encounter with an alien holding a wand – all of these details suggest that the experienced took place in the physical world, and that it not only involved Strieber but every other person who was staying in the cabin that night. (Which is not to imply that everyone in the cabin had a close encounter experience. Strieber certainly did, and his son may have also.)

SP attacks occur on an astral level – which means, of course, that the entity responsible for the attack is a denizen of the astral realm and, generally speaking, is entirely confined to that realm (poltergeist disturbances being an exception). This means that when the SP sufferer wakes up, thereby leaving the astral realm and entering back into the physical realm, they're entirely safe (ostensibly at least); they've left the danger behind. On the other hand, alien abduction episodes occur on a physical level, or quasi-physical level. These beings are able to make a physical manifestation into our realm, grab someone out of bed in the dead of night, transport them to their own realm, and then later return them to the physical realm. To quote from Strieber: "The visitors are physically real. They also function on a non-physical level, and this may be their primary reality."

Although Strieber's October 4 encounter does not sound at all like an

SP attack, some of his other experiences do and could quite possibly be explained as such. If we can accept that some SP episodes involve contact and communication with spirits, it wouldn't be a stretch to imagine that the visitors, able to operate on a non-physical level, make their presence known during SP attacks also. Remember that Strieber said that his interactions with the visitors now take place on a mental level, and that he's basically in telepathic communication with them.

In Strieber's online journal entry for March 12, 2004, he describes a fascinating visitor encounter – similar in nature to an SP episode – which occurred sometime after midnight, while he and Anne were staying at a hotel in Marathon, Texas. Strieber says he remembered hearing the alien presence open the door as it entered the hotel room and that Anne did too. He also recalls being touched by the entity, which he describes as "more of a concentration of awareness than a physical being." He writes: "It was a physical touch, the placing of thin, cool, electric hands on my cheeks. *It was also soul touch, mind touch, even a physical penetration into my organs, my brain*" (my emphasis).

The following morning, says Strieber, "I felt much larger, as if my awareness had expanded to any size I wished…I could hear people thinking…In this state, you not only hear their verbalized thoughts, you see the secret of their essence and in an instant, just at a glance, gain the most intimate knowledge of them." Strieber attributes this heightened state of awareness – this "opening of his third eye" – to the visitor encounter he had had the night before. It was, he says, a "side effect" of the experience, and an undesirable one at that, describing it as "an intrusion on the soul privacy of others."

While driving through Bracketville, Texas, on their way towards San Antonio, Strieber and Anne encountered a police trooper. He describes how he felt at the time: "I really don't like to be near people like policemen and criminals or people with sexual perversions when I'm like this, and this was a man who could have been, were he not holding himself in frantic check, a sex criminal. Souls have an odor, which is why people report scents in the presence of ghosts. Most of them do not smell very well, and this one reeked like sour flowers."

Strieber's heightened state of awareness soon faded. But his mention that "souls have an odor" strikes me interesting because I've noticed the same thing during SP episodes. I explained previously that the SP state allows a person access to a superconscious level of mind – a state of mind in which you are extremely sensitive to the psychic radiation emitted by others, enabling you to "taste" the minds of non-physical beings. That SP episodes take place on an astral level, whereby the soul is exposed and vulnerable, can explain this effect, this increase in psychic sensitivity. Following his visitor encounter, Strieber was clearly operating – as is the SP sufferer during an episode – in a state of total-soul awareness.

Apparently, as a "side effect" of being an abductee, a person's psychic abilities, previously dormant, become active. Strieber has frequent paranormal and mystical experiences, such as OBEs, which he attributes to being in close contact with the visitors. *Transformation* details a number of OBEs almost as spectacular as the ones described by Monroe in *Journeys*. But more on those later.

On July 18, 1986, says Strieber, he experienced something far more spectacular than a simple OBE – he actually levitated. Immediately after lying down in bed to go to sleep, he heard a rustling sound around him, "as if the sheets were still settling." The next thing he knew, he was floating against the ceiling, looking down on the bed. He could clearly see his wife, but the space beside her, where he slept, was empty. He thought he could sense the presence of people nearby, yet was unable to see anyone. His body was paralyzed. "A short time later," he says, "I went spiraling down to the bed, moving through the air quickly and landing softly." Before he was able to tell his wife what had just happened, Strieber quickly fell asleep.

What occurred the following morning is almost as strange as the levitation incident itself. Strieber discovered that when he was asked a question, he would hear a voice "very distinct, beside my right ear, which would give answers." Strieber received the impression that the voice belonged to the visitors. When Anne asked the question "Why did you come here?" the voice cryptically replied, "We saw a glow."

The rest of the questions and answers follow:

"Anne: 'Why are you doing this to Whitley?'

Voice: 'It is time.'

Anne: 'Where are you from?'

Voice: 'Everywhere.'

Anne: 'What's the earth?'

Voice: 'It's a school.'"

After this, says Strieber, the voice took on a completely different quality. "No longer was it a distinct sound, heard as if it were coming from a small speaker just to the right of my head. It became much more thought-like. I suspect that it was very much like what some people hear when they channel." The importance of these words cannot have escaped the reader's attention. That Strieber heard the visitors (or a visitor) in the same two ways that, according to *The Mediums' Book*, a person is able to perceive "spirit sounds" is nothing short of remarkable. It would seem that spirits and so-called alien beings are not all that dissimilar.

It's interesting to note that Strieber's visitors share much in common with the supposedly advanced entities described by Monroe in *Far Journeys*. As the reader may recall, Monroe discovered that, using some kind of "soul technology," these beings are able to affect the astral body, such as by removing it from the physical body. Amazingly, according to Strieber, the visitors are also able to "affect the soul, even draw it out of the body, with technology that may possibly involve the use of high-intensity magnetic fields." Another similarity is that the visitors, like the entities described by Monroe, are able to speak through a human being – although perhaps this is something all non-physical beings are able to do.

In *Transformation*, Strieber describes a visitor experience that occurred in 1986, in which he was sitting downstairs late at night, reading a book on quantum physics, when from the other side of the cabin came nine loud knocks, "in three groups of three, followed by a tenth lighter double knock that communicated an impression of finality." Strieber says the knocks could not have been produced by ordinary human means but formed a cryptic message from the visitors. On the other hand, perhaps what he heard were meaningless "spirit raps," such as the kind that commonly occur in poltergeist disturbances. Are the visitors nothing more than clever, mischievous spirits, posing as alien beings?

Transformation is full of incidents in which Strieber describes hearing a disembodied voice – a voice he attributes to the visitors. On the night of June 13, 1986, for instance, while flicking through the TV channels, Strieber came across a strange program on a public access cable channel. He was initially unsure what the program was about and had no idea what he was looking at. "Then it dawned on me that I was looking at a gruesome act of sexual perversity involving torture." He then heard a voice in his right ear, which said, "We don't like that!" Next, the television switched off inexplicably. This was not due to a power failure, says Strieber, nor was it due to the remote being activated. It was as though the TV had been switched off at the mains. How it happened remains a mystery.

A similar incident occurred on September 12, 1986, says Strieber. On that day, while walking through the woods near his home with his wife, son, and younger brother, Strieber had been feeling rather pleased with his achievements as an author, and the fact that he'd managed to buy such a pleasant property in the country. He admits that he may have behaved in a boastful manner to his brother. All of a sudden he heard a voice – presumably externally – which uttered the words, "Arrogance! I can do what I wish to you." Strieber was so startled by the voice that he "literally jumped out of my skin." He describes it as "loud, very old, and low." No one else heard it. Before returning to the cabin, they all spotted a UFO.

Later in *Transformation*, Strieber provides an explanation as to how these disembodied voices might be produced by the visitors – or indeed anyone, for that matter. First, though, let us look more closely at Strieber's OBEs. Early one morning at around 4:30, Strieber woke up and decided to try for an OBE. He had been reading the work of Monroe, so he knew that he needed to achieve a mind awake/body asleep state. First he saw an image in his mind, "as if on a television screen about a foot from my face." The image was of a visitor – its hand, to be exact – pointing at a box on the floor. For some reason, even though he didn't find the image at all sexually appealing, it "had the effect of causing an explosive sexual reaction in me." Many OBEers, Monroe included, have claimed that the OBE state can bring about strong sexual feelings.

Due to this "blast of sexual energy," Strieber's astral body became loose, and he was able to roll out of his physical body with ease. He floated up into the air, hovering above his physical body, and immediately noticed a cat, lying on the bed, which he realized was one of his own, and which, he ascertained, was in an OBE state, as his cats were (physically) in the city at that time. He also spotted a visitor staring through the window. It looked as if it were guarding it, so he decided to exit the cabin via a different window and found that he could pass straight through the glass and screen. Hovering outside the building, Strieber noticed something strange about the power lines; in his own words – they "appeared fat because of a sort of gray, hairy substance that was adhering to them." He noticed this strange "hairy substance" around the phone line too. "I think that I may have been seeing the electromagnetic field around the wires," he concludes. As the reader may recall, Monroe, while in the OBE state, observed a similar effect in the presence of EM fields.

Shortly afterwards, Strieber entered his body through what appeared to be "an invisible opening," but instead of "waking up," he popped out again and "drifted like a leaf to the floor." He then found himself in his old family home in San Antonio, Texas. Glancing out the window, he saw his father, mowing the lawn. A split second later, Strieber "shot back into" his body and sat up in bed, feeling entirely fine and not at all as though he had just awoken from a dream. What he experienced could not have been a dream or a hallucination, he claims, partly because it was "so completely grounded in the physical world."

In an attempt to get in touch with his "soul," Strieber received some training at the Monroe Institute and began conducting experiments to see if he could leave his body and visit a friend. If Strieber is to be believed – and I think he is – he became highly proficient at astral projection. In one out-of-body experiment, which took place on the morning of March 15, 1988, Strieber attempted to visit a friend, a writer by the name of Barbara Clayman, whose house was located about a thousand miles from New York. Upon arriving at her house in a non-physical state, he found her lying in bed beside her husband. Both of them were asleep. Because he wished to give Clayman an important message, Strieber "projected" his voice into her ear. He explains: "I do not hear myself when I do this. It is a form of thought. My experience is that *it sounds to the listener like a small speaker or radio in his or her ear* (my emphasis)."

As soon as he started "talking" to her, saying "Barbara, it's Whitley," Clayman became frightened and, as far as Strieber could determine, started yelling. He managed, however, to calm her down. Strieber writes, somewhat cryptically, "I am a leaf in the wind at moments like that, and if her husband woke up, I would not be able to maintain my presence." Fortunately her husband did not wake up, and Strieber was able to give her the information she needed – or so he felt at the time. The next evening, Strieber received a call from Barbara, who told him excitedly that she had seen him during the night, and that he had spoken to her. She had apparently seen his face "hanging before her" and was able to recall every word that he had spoken.

On another occasion Strieber attempted to visit a female friend in Denver. She, like most of his other "targets," had no knowledge whatsoever of his OBE activities. That the experiment had been successful was confirmed in a letter she later sent him, in which she claimed that, one night, she woke up and saw an outline of his face across the other side of the room. As she explains in the letter: "What I saw exactly was the impression of your face wearing the glasses you wear amid the leaves of a plant hanging near the door of my bedroom for about three seconds in the dark. I turned on the light and nothing was there."

How fascinating it is to think that these nighttime visitations, which involved both auditory and visual perceptions, would commonly be interpreted as nothing more than hypnagogic/hypnopompic hallucinations, or perhaps SP experiences, when they were in fact encounters between a sleeping person and someone in the OBE state. The same applies, of course, to Monroe's astral visits to R.W., mentioned in the previous chapter. These experiences seem to suggest that the so-called hallucinations experienced by SP sufferers are, in fact, "astral perceptions" and therefore possess a high degree of objectivity. We have found yet more evidence to support the central hypothesis of this book – that some SP attacks are caused by, and involve contact with, discarnate entities.

CHAPTER 17

Trevor James Constable: Etheric Organism Pioneer

These days, photographs of "spirit orbs," UFOs, and other mysterious objects, organisms, and entities, are now quite common due to the widespread use of digital cameras – some of which are sensitive to infrared light (that is, those that aren't equipped with "infrared blockers"). Some of these photographs, I admit, particularly those of spirit orbs, are of a highly dubious nature and can easily be explained away. Indeed many and perhaps most images of orbs are due to distortions of various kinds, caused by the presence of dust particles. You can verify this yourself by conducting a series of simple experiments. Try taking photographs at night, for instance, in a dusty, damp room, with the flash turned on. Orbs aplenty will appear.

I feel it is necessary to address the subject of "paranormal photography" because I believe that, by making advancements in this area, the presence of spirits in our environment will no longer be an issue of debate. We will know for certain that spirits exist all around us, interacting with us, influencing us, causing both harm and benefit. Perhaps we will discover that SP sufferers attract spirits far more than most, in the same way that bright lights draw swarms of insects at night. If clear photographs of spirits interacting with people in the SP state can be obtained, no longer will it be acceptable for the so called experts to classify these experiences as neurological glitches.

What follows next is a brief overview of the revolutionary findings of Trevor James Constable. His research, although primarily focused on the biological UFO phenomenon, is applicable to other living (and non-living) things as well – things which, in his words, "have their main existence in a density that is invisible to human beings of normal vision." And this, of course, includes spirits – not only UFOs. The fact that I've included UFOs and spirits in the same sentence, even compared them to some extent, might strike the reader as ludicrous. As we press forward, however, the connection between these two seemingly separate phenomena will become apparent.

Trevor James Constable was born in New Zealand in 1925. After completing high school, he joined the New Zealand Merchant Marine, followed by the British Merchant Marine. In 1952, he immigrated to the United States, where he still lives today. For twenty-six years he served with the U.S. Merchant Marine, working as a radio electronics officer. During his long career at sea – which spanned almost fifty years – Constable spent much of his free time out on the deck, conducting weather manipulation experiments with a cloudbuster, an orgone energy device invented by the late Dr. Wilhelm Reich. I will briefly describe this technology later.

An aviation and military historian of great note, Constable has written – on his own and in collaboration with other authors – a number of classic books on fighter aviation, by far the most popular being *The Blood Knight of Germany* (1970), an official biography of the world's greatest fighter ace Erich Hartmann. His first book on the topic of UFOs, *They Live in the Sky*, was published in 1958 and is considered a rare classic. This was followed, in 1976, by his masterwork, *The Cosmic Pulse of Life: The Revolutionary Biological Power Behind UFOs*. The latter is basically an expanded version of the former, containing additional findings.

Constable developed an interest in UFOlogy during the 1950s, when the "contactee" phenomenon was in full swing, and people like George Adamski, Truman Bethurum, Orfeo Angelucci and others claimed to be in communication with benevolent "space brothers." As a young man, Constable had formed the opinion that UFO occupants, instead of using radio like us, were bound to be making use of a far more advanced means of communication, such as telepathy.

Constable is a communications expert of sorts, having worked in his teens as a staff writer for radio programs in New Zealand, as a radio actor, as well as a shipboard radio operator. In an attempt to find out more about UFO communication methods, Constable began learning as much as he could about the contactees and their teachings. Many of the contactees were genuine mediums – which meant, of course, that the means by which they received information from their respective "UFO sources" involved telepathy in some shape or form.

Constable became acquainted with who is now one of the most famous and respected contactees of all time – George Van Tassel (1910-1978), also known as the "Sage of Giant Rock." An aircraft mechanic and flight inspector, Van Tassel lived in the desert of Southern California and had built his home around Giant Rock, the largest freestanding boulder in the world. Beside the rock, Van Tassel had also set up a restaurant, as well the facilities for his annual spacecraft convention. A chamber had been hewn out of the ground beneath the giant rock, and it was in this space that Van Tassel held regular channeling sessions with the Council of Seven Lights, a supposed body of discarnate Earthlings inhabiting a spaceship orbiting our planet. Constable began attending these communication sessions and was greatly impressed by what he witnessed. At a typical session, he says, around sixty to seventy people would show up, including college professors and reputable businessmen.

The first stage of these séance type gatherings – called by Constable the "call phase" – involved chanting and singing songs, so as to attract the attention of the UFO intelligences with whom they desired to communicate. "The call phase is intended to stand out above the psychic background noise as a strong radio signal does above radio noise and weaker stations," explains Constable. For the "call phase" to be successful, he says, Van Tassel was required to function as a "psychic radio operator," focusing "the power of his transmitter"– "the biological energies of his gathering" – in a very specific way, so that the UFO intelligences would receive his "signal" and thus respond accordingly. And respond they did. Within moments, an entity would proceed to speak through Van Tassel. Immediately after it had finished, another entity would speak, then another.

Being a former radio actor, Constable knew a lot about voice and speech and had mastered the techniques by which radio actors and announcers are able to change their voice when playing different characters in a radio play. Because, according to Constable, Van Tassel was able to achieve, using his voice, feats that even the greatest radio actors would be unable to accomplish, he could not have been using trickery and was definitely a genuine medium. When the various intelligences spoke through him, says Constable, "there was in each case a distinct change of the speech pattern, pace, voice timbre, accent and subject matter. No radio actor could have done it."

But there was yet another reason Constable knew the voices were genuine. About a split second before they issued from Van Tassels's mouth, Constable was able to hear, in his head, the thoughts of the particular UFO entity who was speaking at the time. As a result, Constable "knew what Van Tassel was going to say before he got it out as audible sound." Constable was greatly surprised by this phenomenon. Prior to its occurrence, he knew almost nothing about psychic phenomena and was totally inexperienced in this area.

Without being aware of the dangers involved, Constable, wanting to become a medium for UFO intelligences himself, asked Van Tassel how he should go about it. Happy to help, Van Tassel gave him certain routines to follow, which Constable practiced with "diligence and persistence." Van Tassel's instructions must have worked, because, on one occasion, for a short moment, Constable became a "loudspeaker" for UFO intelligences. Over time, he became extremely sensitive to such communications – too sensitive, in fact. This caused problems. His mind was constantly bombarded by bits and pieces of information, most of it "confusing rubbish."

Furthermore, he unintentionally developed the capacity to read the minds of other people and was often aware of what other people were thinking, and what they were about to say, before they had a chance to open their mouth. Constable became psychic in other ways, too. Whenever the phone rang, for instance, he instantly knew who was on the other end of the line prior to picking up the handset. He also claims that UFOs would manifest in his presence after promising to do so, and that on one occasion he witnessed a group of luminous UFOs being intercepted by military aircraft from a nearby base.

In *The Cosmic Pulse*, Constable explains the extent of his troubles: "A constant struggle soon ensued for control of my physical vehicle – myself against unseen interlopers. I was fighting continually against various forms of automatism... My difficulties were extreme, and I felt that I was slowly losing my battle to retain my mastery of myself. I bitterly regretted ever having meddled in UFO communications. The 'intelligences' into whose realm I had broken poured confusing rubbish into me."

Those with no understanding of spirit possession and the like would probably make the assumption that Constable had developed schizophrenia, accompanied by auditory hallucinations. Thankfully, the readers of this book know better. As a result of practicing Van Tassel's "psychic development" exercises in an attempt to gain mediumistic powers, Constable opened himself up to possession by troublesome discarnate entities. As to whether or not the entities he was in communication with were in fact "UFO intelligences" – and this applies to Van Tassel as well – is difficult to say. To me they sound a lot like lower astral entities. This is a moot point, however, and shouldn't greatly concern us at the present.

Just when he thought the voices in his head were about to drive him permanently crazy, Constable became acquainted with a highly accomplished occultist named Franklin Thomas, who was more than willing to help him with his problem. As well as being the owner of a new age publishing company, Thomas ran his own bookstore where he gave lectures on esoteric topics. "This shabby little man had conscious control of the hidden forces of nature, and he wielded his power in setting me free," explains Constable. Assisted by Thomas, and within a very short period of time, Constable managed to suppress his mediumistic powers entirely. Thomas instructed him to suppress his other psychic abilities as well, explaining that it needed to be done for the sake of genuine spiritual growth. Constable complied. He was told that one of his missions in life was to help solve the UFO mystery, and that being involved with "psychic forces" would only lead to his downfall and cause him to stray from a much truer path.

Unlike van Tassel – the "psychic radio operator" – Constable had become little more than a "psychic radio receiver" that could not be switched off. During this time, though, he did in fact receive some valuable information about UFOs; not all of it was "confusing rubbish." In a conversation he had with Thomas, Constable was told "that those intelligences which would seek to communicate *without controlling* [my emphasis] had what seemed to be the valid information." The Spiritists, I'm sure, would agree with this statement.

As concerns the valuable – and highly unconventional – UFO information that Constable received telepathically, a few main points are worth listing: 1. "UFOs are space ships, but their vibratory makeup is not fixed in the physical-material density. They are *mutants*." 2. "There are normally-invisible living things in space that are *not* space ships." 3. "Infrared film, exposed between dawn and sunrise in high, dry locales will frequently objectify invisible objects of various kinds living in and passing through the atmosphere."

Working from little more information than this, Constable, together with a friend named James O. Woods, set about trying to test if UFOs could indeed be photographed with infrared film. Beginning in the late 1950s, the majority of their photographic work took place in the high desert of California – apparently an ideal environment in which to photograph invisible UFOs. Constable and Woods used cameras that were nothing special or remarkable. In *The Cosmic Pulse*, Constable recommends using a simple analogue camera – preferably one with a good lens. The camera must be fitted with an 87 filter and infrared film. Treated with special dyes, infrared – "heat sensitive" – film is sensitive to the infrared portion of the electromagnetic spectrum. As for the 87 filter, this allows *only* infrared light to pass through the lens of the camera.

The term "infrared" is basically a scientific name for heat. All objects above the temperature of absolute zero absorb and emit infrared radiation. Even ice cubes emit infrared radiation. Infrared light (or radiation), which lies between the visible and microwave portions of the electromagnetic spectrum, exists in two main forms – near infrared and far infrared. Near infrared, which is closest in wavelength to visible light, is non-thermal and cannot be felt. The sensors on TV remotes make use of this type of infrared light.

Far infrared, on the other hand, is closer to the microwave region of the electromagnetic spectrum and is therefore thermal. We experience it every day in the form of heat, such as when we sit in front of the fire or when we expose ourselves to sunlight. As an object slowly heats up – such as a piece of coal in a fire, for example – it will begin to emit infrared radiation. Initially, while the object is still black, most of the energy it emits will be in the form of heat. As the temperature of the object increases, it will begin to glow red, therefore emitting visible light. The warmer the object, the more infrared radiation it will emit.

According to Constable, a correlation exists between the development of radar prior to World War II – and its subsequent widespread use – and the modern advent of UFOs, which started, of course, with Kenneth Arnold's famous 1947 sighting of nine unusual objects flying in a chain formation near Mt. Rainier, Washington. Arnold concluded, by the way, that UFOs "...are groups and masses of living organisms that are as much a part of our atmosphere and space as the life we find in the oceans." For those who don't know, radar detects objects using high frequency radio pulses, which bounce off the objects they strike; with the return signal, the object can be tracked. In a sense, radar is able to feel electronically for objects that cannot be seen with the naked eye. It should be noted, furthermore, that the infrared portion of the electromagnetic spectrum adjoins the microwave portion of the spectrum, while radar basically consists of pulsed microwave energy.

With the widespread use of radar for wartime purposes, a large number of invisible, airborne objects were detected by the military – objects which, once "intercepted," were sometimes found not to exist. They were nicknamed "angels," among other things, and they continued to show up on military radar screens. Those who saw them were astonished by the fact that they could materialize and dematerialize almost instantaneously, travel incredible speeds, and achieve maneuvers that not even dragonflies would be capable of.

Some of these objects were biological in nature, says Constable, and would not have suddenly appeared in the dramatic fashion they did had the ether not been disturbed by so much harmful microwave energy. The widespread use of radar transformed the planet into a "veritable electromagnetic hedgehog," he says. Constable mentions the fact that pulsed electromagnetic energies – such as radar – can penetrate one's body, causing heating of the skin and nerve endings, eye damage, and coagulation of body proteins. If indeed some UFOs are living creatures – and, like us, can be harmed by microwave energy – this might explain why they're sometimes observed to glow in the night sky.

To attract biological UFOs (or "critters," as he also calls them) to his vicinity, so that they could be photographed, Constable would perform a simple, esoteric procedure called the "star exercise," which supposedly had the effect of energizing and enlarging his etheric body, turning him into a "bioenergetic beacon." Apparently, out in the desert, on a very dry day, Woods was able to perceive Constable's etheric body – "a huge, luminous sphere that pulsed regularly with my movements." The more he repeated the exercise, the larger his etheric body would grow. At times, he says, its diameter would extend to a distance of more than one hundred feet!

Standing some distance away, Woods would attempt to photograph the "blindingly fast flashes of movement" that could occasionally be seen around Constable's body. Constable, meanwhile, was also able to perceive these luminous flashes. If Constable and Woods were lucky, these elusive beings would show up on film, the majority of which were found to be bell-shaped, resembling the bell-shaped flying discs commonly reported by witnesses. Over many years of traveling out to the desert and taking infrared photographs in this fashion during the pre-dawn hours, Constable and Woods managed to obtain some quite remarkable images of biological UFOs. These organisms, concluded Constable, are essentially plasmatic, "having their form expressed in heat substance. They travel in pulsatory fashion, swelling and shrinking cyclically as they move through the air, much as we pulsate with our heartbeat and swell and shrink with our lung movements."

In his classic book *Supernature*, the late Lyall Watson devotes a section to the aura, which, he suggests, could be electromagnetic in nature, possibly plasmatic. Our bodies, he says, send out electromagnetic waves just beyond the range of the visible spectrum, which is that portion of the electromagnetic spectrum that can be perceived by the human eye, lying between 380 and 760 millimicrons (mm). "Those who claim to be able to see an aura surrounding living things," he explains, "could be supersensitive to the infrared end of the spectrum." Infrared radiation has wavelengths between about 750 nm and 1 mm. Animals with good night vision, such as owls, have some sensitivity to infrared radiation put out by their prey, says Watson. He cites an experiment in which owls, although able to detect a silent mouse from some distance away, were unable to locate a piece of dead meat of the same size and shape no matter how close.

Constable claims to have photographed etheric organisms of many different varieties, some small, others monstrously large. Not all of them were bell-shaped. He lists them as "great spherical critters that looked like atmospheric jellyfish," "fish like forms," "serpents," and "elementals of various kinds." As for serpents, Constable says he managed to photograph such a creature, not out in the desert, but in a populated city environment. The two photographs he took of the beast – taken using high-speed infrared film – showed it curled up beside a telephone pole. "This etheric monster had its head curled around toward me, and in one exposure I was photographing through perhaps six or eight feet of his body lying directly behind his head."

Because these entities have "their main existence in a density that is invisible to human beings of normal vision," it's not surprising that the majority of UFO photographs taken by Constable show subtle, ghostly forms. By altering their vibratory makeup, he says, these organisms are able to materialize in our dimension at times of their choosing. When this occurs, (which is obviously very infrequently) they can be seen with the naked eye and are often thought to be spaceships from other planets. To photograph materialized UFOs, infrared film would not be required. The only reason Constable used infrared film is because what he was trying to photograph – and indeed managed to photograph – were UFOs in their natural, invisible state.

To illustrate how a UFO is able to alter its vibratory makeup and either enter or leave our dimension, Constable uses the example of an electric fan. When the fan is turning at full speed, all one sees is a blur; the blades are almost invisible. However, when the fan is switched to a lower setting, its individual blades can easily be discerned. What has occurred is a lowering of frequency. According to occult thought, because the astral realm (or the etheric realm, for that matter) exists on a higher frequency than our own, its denizens therefore operate on a higher frequency to us, preventing us from ever making full physical contact with them. Our realm and their realm are "out of synch." Even so, the two realms, instead of being separated like rooms in a house, blend into each other, much like colors in a sunset.

The reason why spirits, gray aliens, and other paranormal entities remain so elusive is because they have their main existence in another realm, and because they have a limited ability to materialize in our realm. Despite this, their ability to influence and manipulate incarnates is extremely strong and should not be underestimated. The school bully who is too small and weak to scare the other children inflicts not physical abuse but verbal abuse. He uses his mind to cause harm, and the mind is far more powerful than a fist. Similarly, malevolent spirits and other beings of this nature, being unable to influence us overtly and physically, rely, instead, on psychic means. Like a deadly cancer, they secretly attack us from the inside.

In *The Cosmic Pulse*, Constable devotes several chapters to the subject of psychic mind control and the malevolent excarnate beings who use such tactics, whom he calls "the boys downstairs" and whom he believes are behind some of the more negative UFO encounters, such as those that have resulted in the death of Air Force pilots. As for the "cosmic good guys" – the opposing force to the boys downstairs – Constable refers to them as "the etherians." There is, he says, "a war in progress for the mind of man," involving these two spiritual forces.

When he first set out to photograph UFOs, admits Constable, he was hoping to find spaceships but instead found living creatures. Initially this was something of a disappointment. He eventually recognized, however, that many of us are resistant to the idea of biological UFOs because "what is alive in UFOs stimulates through resonance and correspondence that which is alive in man. He cannot stand this movement." The Austrian-American psychiatrist, psychoanalyst, and scientist Wilhelm Reich (1897-1957), whose research Constable discusses in *The Cosmic Pulse*, named this neurotic, anti-life attitude – this inability to confront life – "armoring." Reich defined "armoring" as "a negative attitude towards life and sex..."

In time, UFOs that were not biological but were clearly structured, engineered craft, began to appear on Constable's infrared photographs. He called them "ether ships." These objects, he says, are powered by orgone energy, which is utilized in such a way as to produce a whirling force field around the craft. He speculates that these force fields might create plasmas and would explain why some people receive severe burns while in close contact with UFOs. Fascinating though this research is, it's the biological side of Constable's work that concerns us the most. And it is this topic to which we will now return.

Not only has Constable photographed critters, he has also filmed them. Included in *The Cosmic Pulse* are six incredible frames, excerpted from infrared motion picture footage, showing "bioforms" swarming in the air above Constable's head. The sequence was shot at twenty four frames per second, while the event of the bioforms in motion occurred extremely quickly – within a quarter of a second, to be exact – suggesting that they move at lightning fast speeds. The bioforms in the film are shown changing shape, position, and dividing like amoebae. The resemblance of these creatures to amoebae and other unicellular micro-organisms is extremely striking. Because of their appearance and behavior, Constable concluded that biological UFOs are fairly simple life forms, possessed of a rudimentary intelligence.

In *The Cosmic Pulse*, much information is given on the topic of orgone energy – Reich's name for etheric energy – and Constable reveals how the properties of this energy shed light on the UFO mystery. Biological UFOs, he asserts, are etheric energy beings, "living in an ocean of living energy," while ether ships, as already discussed, utilize this energy as a means of propulsion. Orgone energy – sometimes referred to as "cosmic life energy" – is said to exist in free form in the atmosphere and also in the vacuum of space. And, although it is not electromagnetic in nature itself, it constitutes the medium through which all electromagnetic disturbances are transmitted. As a result, the orgone has often been called, or likened to, "the ether."

"Orgone energy functions appear across the whole of creation, in microbes, storm clouds, hurricanes and galaxies. It not only charges and animates the natural world, we are immersed in a sea of it, much as a fish is immersed in water," explains James DeMeo in his illuminating book *The Orgone Energy Accumulator Handbook*. "In addition, it is the medium which communicates emotion and perception, through which we are connected to the cosmos, and made kin with all that is living."

Constable retired from UFO research in 1979, and now spends much of his time conducting weather-engineering projects for governments. These projects involve the use of Reich's aforementioned cloudbuster – a device that is able to manipulate the orgone energy potentials in the atmosphere, allowing the operator to control the weather and, more importantly, combat environmental destruction. It can apparently be used to dissipate smog in highly polluted areas and to produce rain in drought affected areas. At present, Constable is the chief consultant of a company based in Singapore called Etheric Rain Engineering Pte. Ltd. So far, the company's smog dissipation projects – such as "Checker," "Breakthrough," and "Victor" – have been highly successful. The cloudbuster played an important part in Constable's UFO research, or more specifically, his ability to photograph UFOs. Using this device with skill and precision, he was able to attract critters to his immediate vicinity so that they could be photographed. No longer was he required to perform the "star exercise."

Reich's experiments with orgone energy led him to construct a device called an "orgone energy accumulator," which, as its name suggests, accumulates orgone energy. It consists of a box lined with alternating layers of organic and inorganic materials, which serve to either absorb or reflect this energy. Orgone energy is drawn inside the box, where it remains trapped in a highly concentrated form. According to some, including Constable, this device can be used to verify one of Reich's discoveries – that high concentrations of orgone energy, such as that produced by the accumulator, desensitize film emulsions, creating dark areas on photographs. Constable's photographic work bears this out, particularly with regards to his photographs of ether ships. "What we saw as bright streaks to our extended vision, turned out to be black on the finished prints," he explains.

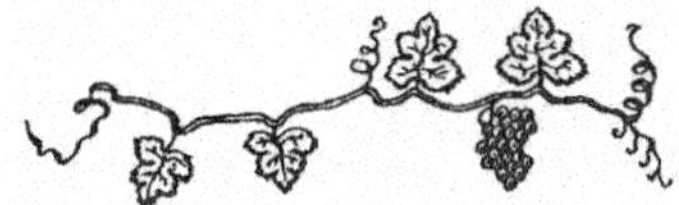

In the late 1970s, following the publication of *The Cosmic Pulse*, Constable received an exciting letter from a UFO researcher in Genoa, Italy, by the name of Signor Luciano Boccone. The late Boccone, who worked as an executive with a metals fabricating company, explained to Constable how he and his team of researchers had managed to obtain, independently of Constable, identical photographs of biological UFOs. Not only that, explained Boccone, but a Romanian friend of his by the name of Florin Gheorghita independently substantiated Constable's findings as well. The work of all three researchers – Constable, Boccone, and Gheorghita – is practically identical, meaning that many of the lifeforms they photographed are exactly the same in appearance and behavior.

When Boccone and his colleagues first began their investigation into invisible UFOs in 1976, they knew absolutely nothing of Constable or his work. Their UFO research group, run by Boccone, was composed of some twenty-five members, most of them highly educated, holding degrees in science and engineering. (Whether or not the group still exists is difficult to determine.) Because they were ignorant of orgone energy and the like, the methods they developed to photograph invisible UFOs were completely different from Constable's. Nevertheless, they managed to obtain some very impressive results, as evidenced by their photographs.

To detect the presence of invisible UFOs in their vicinity so that they could be photographed using infrared film (as well as other types of film, such as ultraviolet), Boccone and his colleagues used a variety of electronic instruments, including Geiger counters, magnetic compasses, temperature indicators, and ultrasound and ultraviolet indicators. Boccone gives a rundown of the methods used by his group to photograph UFOs: "As a rule, whenever our instruments warn us of any irregular quick variation in radioactivity and/or magnetic field, air temperature, luminosity, etc., we take immediate pictures in the same direction in which such variations are detected." Boccone adds that the appearance of an invisible UFO usually results in a high Geiger counter reading – of around 0.2 mR/h and above – as well as compass needle deflections. Sometimes, too, other instruments will "go crazy" for no apparent reason.

In his letter to Constable, Boccone wrote: "Like your own files and Gheorghita's, our records are full of photographs showing invisible, glowing, pulsating plasmaorganisms, capable of changing shape, size, density, luminosity, arrangement, position, etc, in a split second…They show invisible plasmatic bodies fleeing or cavorting in the sky at tremendous speed, or hovering or 'dancing' over our research areas. When they also land sometimes, in the form of invisible spheres of light which subsequently transmute in a fraction of a second either into invisible, glowing, seemingly-ectoplasmic, demon-like entities, or into invisible 'arabesques of light' skimming over the ground, or into invisible, yet corporeal, haloed human-like entities. Or where they also show up sometimes, in the form of invisible, small light balls, cavorting around us or creeping up to us, seemingly going their rounds before taking off."

Like Constable, Boccone was of the opinion that the majority of UFOs seen in our skies are not alien spacecraft at all, but rather "generally invisible, ultra-dimensional, ultra-terrestrial, biological, etheric organisms that are of our planet, that have been living with us, side by side, unnoticed since the beginning of time." Boccone died suddenly and unexpectedly in 1981 from an infarct, but not before he'd spent some time conducting UFO research with Constable – clearly his hero – who taught him how to build and operate various orgone devices, such as the cloudbuster. Using this technology presumably allowed Boccone and his colleagues to advance their UFO research.

No doubt the reader will have recognized by now that an explicit overlap exists between the UFO phenomenon and what one might term the "discarnate entity phenomenon." As Constable's and Boccone's UFO research illustrates, there is no fine line between UFO entities and spirits. I direct the reader's attention in particular to the "invisible, glowing, seemingly-ectoplasmic, demon-like entities," and the "invisible, yet corporeal, haloed human-like entities," that were allegedly photographed by Boccone and his colleagues. These sound a lot like spirits to me – not UFO entities.

Could some of them be the spirits of the dead, I wonder? Or OBEers going about their business? Or perhaps elementals? When I first came across Boccone's colorful description of these entities, which reads like something out of a science-fiction or fantasy novel, I was immediately struck by his mentioning of "invisible balls of light" and "small light balls" and the like, as I have seen, while in the hypnopompic state, "spirit orbs" floating around my bedroom that are similar in appearance to some of the "orbs" that appear in photographs taken by digital cameras

Those familiar with "ghost hunting" techniques would have noticed that many of the same electronic instruments used by Boccone and his colleagues to detect biological UFOs are also employed by "ghost hunters" to find spirits in supposedly haunted locations. In almost every environment of paranormal activity involving non-physical entities, either in a haunted house or a place where alien abductions have taken place – such as Strieber's cabin, for example – electronic devices are known to behave in odd ways for no apparent reason.

Pondering these matters further, I began to wonder if Boccone's "invisible entity detection methods," involving the use of Geiger counters and magnetic compasses and the like, could be used to combat SP attacks by alerting the SP sufferer of the sudden appearance of potentially harmful discarnate entities. If, or when, these devices "go crazy," it could trigger an alarm of some sort, waking the sleeper up before an SP attack is about to occur. Perhaps, too, the system could be connected to an infrared camera – either a still camera or video camera – enabling one to obtain photographs or video footage of spirits. I have long wondered if SP sufferers – perhaps because their auras are unique and stand out – attract the attention of spirits more so than non-SP sufferers, much in the same way that a man with a gangrenous wound is likely to attract more flies than a man who's perfectly healthy. Because of this hypothetical ability to draw spirits, it might be easy to photograph, at night, spirits surrounding the bodies of SP sufferers. These are all interesting possibilities.

CHAPTER 18

Postscript

During the many challenging months it's taken me to write and research this book, my opinion of the SP phenomenon – and indeed my opinion of my own SP experiences – has changed markedly, shifting from a largely negative viewpoint to a very positive one. This came about through having realized that the SP state is doorway to many possibilities, some terrifying, some interesting and delightful, others simply weird and baffling. Overall, I think the condition is a gift – a tool, which, when used properly, can be immensely rewarding.

During the month of April 2008, I made a conscious decision to face my fear of the SP phenomenon. I would try, I decided, to experiment a little with the condition, to see if I could gain something new from it. I wanted, in particular, to use the SP state as a means of experiencing LDs and OBEs. To undergo a LD while in the SP state, Conesa recommends breathing calmly and focusing one's attention on one's navel area. Top of the list, however, was my desire to have an OBE.

I decided that, instead of waiting for an SP attack to occur spontaneously – and then trying for an OBE or LD – I would attempt to induce the SP state. In other words, *I would make myself have an SP episode*. But, I worried, would this be playing with fire? Would I be making myself a candidate for spirit possession? Should I really be fooling around with altered states of consciousness? All of these concerns – and more – were weighing heavily on my mind. I decided, in the end, that I was probably being paranoid. And anyway, I thought, nothing ventured, nothing gained.

In William Buhlman's highly readable *Adventures Beyond the Body*, the author lists numerous techniques on how to induce an OBE, one of the most effective being what he calls "the early morning technique." To do this, he says, you must set your alarm before going to bed, so that you wake up very early in the morning, after two or three REM periods – around three to five hours – have passed. Once awake – but obviously not fully awake – you should move to another area of the house and lie down. The couch is a perfect option. By relaxing and directing your attention away from your physical body, the hypnagogic state, and hence the SP state, should be quite easy to achieve. From there, OBEs and LDs are within your grasp. "Using this technique, many people report an out-of-body experience immediately after they drift to sleep," writes Buhlman.

To direct your attention away from your body, Buhlman recommends practicing various visualization techniques, one of which involves picturing a room in your mind – not your own bedroom, but the lounge room in your mother's house, for example. You should imagine the room as vividly as possible and become absorbed in its details. The key to this exercise, says Buhlman, "is to maintain your interest outside your body until your body falls asleep." I think that sleeping in another area of your house after waking up is unnecessary and could quite possibly ruin the entire exercise by causing you to wake up too fully. For this reason, whenever I practice this technique, I stay put in bed, attempting to maintain a drowsy state of consciousness.

One night in late April, I woke up at 4:00 a.m., having set my alarm for this time. I had been dreaming prior to this but could no longer remember the exact content of the dream. When I switched off the alarm and lay back down in bed, my mind was still very relaxed, as I hadn't yet woken up completely – which was exactly what I had aimed to do. Entering the hypnagogic state was no easy task, as my mind became occupied by various mundane concerns, such as what the coming day might bring. I was also worried that my SP experiment might fail, and that instead of having an OBE or a LD I would spend the rest of the morning awake, unable to get to sleep, and end up too tired to complete a proper day's work.

About forty minutes later, I managed to enter the hypnagogic state. Within moments, my body became paralyzed and heavy, and I seemed to sink into the bed. I had entered a light SP state. There was, I could tell, an entity nearby. I could feel it sitting on my legs. Its mind had a strong odor, and I could sense it was less than benevolent. This was a carnal, un-evolved creature whose sole reason for showing up was simply to cause me grief. The next thing I knew, the entity, which was still seated on my legs, began rocking back and forth, as though attempting to copulate with me. Or at least that's the impression I received. Whatever action it was trying to perform simply wasn't working. To my intense relief, it soon gave up.

A second later, I felt as though I were floating. I had, by this stage, lost all awareness of lying in bed; my consciousness, you might say, was focused elsewhere. The entity was still with me, and this made me anxious. It grabbed me by the hands and proceeded to drag me down. Our descent went on and on. Strangely, though, I was not as frightened as I thought I would be. In fact, the situation struck me as absurd. Why, I asked myself, was I letting myself fall? Why not try and fly? Feeling empowered, I did just that; I shook the little bastard off and rose into the air like a rocket. The feeling was exhilarating.

The next thing I knew, I was flying through a patch of thick, grey clouds, the weather cold and stormy. Below me was a beach. So beautiful were my surroundings, and so enjoyable and exciting was the experience of being airborne, that I started to become conscious of my body. I was beginning to wake up, and this didn't please me at all. The moment I crashed into the beach, the LD came to an end. I felt disappointed for failing to sustain the experience but at the same time pleased for managing to induce it. My first experiment had been a success.

The experience gave me a taste of what can be achieved by using the SP state as a portal to other "worlds." Perhaps more importantly, though, it made me realize that frightening and unpleasant SP episodes needn't necessarily remain that way, that it's possible to transform these experiences and to benefit greatly as a result. Never have I felt as satisfied as I did at the moment I escaped the clutches of the malevolent entity that was trying to drag me down. A Jungian psychologist would probably interpret this experience – perhaps all of my SP experiences – as confrontations between me and my "shadow," the repressed "alter-ego" of my unconscious mind. That I managed to leave it behind and, in a sense, overcome it, would be seen as a positive thing, I suppose. Or perhaps the complete opposite, because according to Jungian psychology you must face and integrate your shadow self, rather than repress it, and run from it – which seems to have been what I did.

In applying Jung's concept of the shadow to the SP phenomenon, some interesting ideas emerge. In a definition of the shadow written by Hans Dieckmann, we are told: "In dreams and fantasies the shadow appears with the characteristics of a personality of the same sex as the ego, but in a very different configuration. It is presented as the eternal antagonist of an individual or group, or the dark brother within, who always accompanies one, the way Mephistopheles accompanied Goethe's Faust." In my short story, "Beware of the Spirits," written when I knew absolutely nothing about the SP phenomenon or, for that matter, Jungian psychology, I named the vampiric entity that repeatedly attacks me during my sleep "the shadow." Is this just a coincidence? Or did I pluck this name from Jung's "collective unconscious?"

Compelling though my first "SP experiment" was, my second experiment yielded even more spectacular results. It involved either an OBE or an extremely vivid LD. Why I'm not sure if it was the former or the latter will shortly become apparent. On this occasion, little effort was required to reach the SP state, and, fortunately, no spirits were around to cause me any trouble or discomfort, so I was easily able to focus my mind. As I lay on the bed in a state of warm, comfortable paralysis, I could hear various activities going on around me. I initially assumed that these noises were caused by my housemate, that perhaps he had gotten out of bed and gone to the kitchen. As I listened more closely, however, I gradually came to realize that what I was hearing were not normal noises caused by events in the "real world" but what could best be termed "astral noises." I've heard such noises before, but never has the experience lasted so long.

Most of these "astral noises" were of doors shutting and closing, footsteps, and people talking. There seemed to be several people in the house going about their daily routine. In particular, I could hear a man and a woman, both of whom sounded young, having a discussion about domestic matters. Their voices emanated from the direction of the kitchen. Coming from the room beside me – which was unoccupied at the time – were the cries of a baby or young child. I received the impression that the man and the woman were a couple, and that the infant belonged to them. Perhaps, I thought, I was hearing noises from the past – when the house was occupied by a family – noises which, having been recorded in the "psychic ether," were now being picked up by my mind like a radio receiver picking up a station. Which is not to imply, of course, that these noises sounded in any way ghostly or artificial; they sounded entirely real, which is why I initially mistook them for "real" noises.

What followed next was a brief period of light sleep. When I "woke up," I was back in the SP state. A humming sound – like that of a motorcycle engine – filled my head. Realizing that this sound heralded the beginning of an OBE, I encouraged it to increase in volume and frequency, which it did. I then seemed to shoot out from my body, as though propelled by a powerful surge of energy. As I continued to rise higher and higher, I glanced below and was able to discern the lights of the city. A split second later, I was floating in outer space, looking "down" at the Earth. The sight was immensely beautiful. I should mention that everything I saw during this experience, including the Earth, was highly detailed and in full color; it all looked entirely real and life-like.

As expected, I was positioned above Australia and Asia. Because, for some reason, Japan stood out from the other countries I could see, I decided to fly down and take a look. Reaching my destination was almost instantaneous, and I seemed to land with a slight jolt. My astral body, or "dream body," was not entirely weightless. I was standing on what looked like the shore of a lake. The ground was covered in thick, green grass, which went right up to the edge of the water. I decided to sit down and relax. In an experiment to test the reality of the situation – to see if it was a LD or an OBE – I ran my hand along the top of the grass and was actually able to feel it. I also tried placing my foot in the water, but for some reason I was unable to do so. As I started to make my way across the grass and away from the lake, the experience began to transform into a dream, and I gradually woke up. I recall the sensation of falling from a great height and landing in my body. During the course of the night, I kept drifting in and out of the SP state, and therefore got little sleep. The experiment was well worth it though.

I haven't yet conducted any further SP experiments, as I don't feel I'm ready to do so. Compelling though it is to explore the psychic side of your being, it's also incredibly challenging and draining, and, I expect, if you were not cautious about it, could possibly lead to mental imbalance. It's very solitary, too; if you need advice, you has virtually no one to turn to. Given the fact that I have SP episodes on a regular basis as it is, I don't necessary need to experience any more. If you encourage these experiences too much, I think, you might find yourself being consumed by them. Most of us, myself included, find it hard enough dealing with the demands and responsibilities of this world – of earning a living, paying the bills, maintaining friendships, and so on – that, to simultaneously "live" in another world – the "spirit realm" – would be almost impossible.

How individuals like Monroe, Swedenborg, and Fortune managed to keep a foot firmly planted in both worlds, and cope successfully with the challenges of each, is remarkable to say the least. If there is such a thing as spiritual advancement, and as Strieber's visitors claim the earth is a "school" for souls, it's likely that a very small percentage of the population has reached the stage in their "education" where they're able to move beyond the physical realm and explore other worlds. And by this I'm not suggesting that SP sufferers, OBE travelers, and others who regularly have "spiritual" experiences are any more "evolved" than anyone else. I certainly don't claim to be anyone special. In most respects I'm a fairly ordinary man, and although I've always had an interest in paranormal and occult matters, my imagination is no more active than that of the average person. I didn't go looking for spirits; they came looking for me.

Writing this book has been something of a catharsis for me. When

I first starting working on it, most of the SP attacks I had undergone – and was undergoing at the time – were extremely frightening, in that they seemed to involve some element of "psychic attack." During such an experience, you feel as though your mind is being invaded by a malevolent entity. It is, as I said, a kind of rape, and is wholly unpleasant. I'm pleased to say that I haven't undergone one of these "mind invasion" SP attacks in a very long time –and hopefully I won't ever again. I remain convinced that these particular SP attacks are an attempt at possession by malevolent discarnate entities and could quite possibly lead to other types of paranormal phenomena, such as poltergeist disturbances and permanent auditory hallucinations. Let us not forget that spirit possession is a very real phenomenon, which mainly affects those who, because they're stressed, nervous, or depressed, and are therefore leaking vital energy, have rendered themselves psychically vulnerable.

While we're on the topic of SP and mental illness, namely the possibility that SP could lead to the development of something akin to schizophrenia, a few words of warning should be given. The reader will have noticed that I use the word "possibility," and indeed I have chosen this word very carefully, as I do not wish to cause unnecessary alarm to those who suffer from SP. Fearing that as a result of SP you might become a victim of spirit possession, or that you might develop a serious mental illness, is by no means recommended, which is not to imply that these fears are unfounded.

Those who have serious and terrifying SP attacks on a regular basis and experience difficulty coping with the condition might benefit from consulting a health professional who knows about SP, such as a sleep specialist. For that matter, too, they might benefit equally as much, or perhaps more, from consulting a shaman (not that shamans are easy to come by) or even a Spiritist medium. I'm not qualified to offer advice on the matter. There are sadly very few health professionals who know about SP and are accurately able to diagnose the condition and, if necessary, treat it.

David Hufford wisely recommends caution when relating SP to schizophrenia. In an email to me, he wrote: "There is solid research data...that ordinary SP experiencers are at great risk of being diagnosed as schizophrenic. That is tragic." Hufford's right – it is tragic. As an SP sufferer myself, I would not like to be misdiagnosed as schizophrenic, nor would I wish this upon others. It is my sincere hope that this book will bring clarity and understanding to the topic of SP – not the opposite.

In this book, we've explored a number of theories as to what might cause SP episodes. Not all of these theories concern the influence of spirits or are particularly paranormal. Is it possible, I wonder, to come up with a definitive explanation for the phenomenon, one that encompasses all of the others?

When it comes to the study of paranormal phenomena – let's take UFOs as an example – researchers often make the mistake of choosing one particular theory that appeals to them, such as the very limited Extraterrestrial Hypothesis (ETH), and sticking solely to that theory, by acknowledging the evidence that supports it and ignoring the evidence that doesn't. This is easy to do because not only is the UFO phenomenon complex, multi-layered and elusive, but UFOs consist of many different things, some of them contradictory, from intelligent "earth lights" to possible craft from other planets, or other "realities."

All of these explanations must be taken into consideration – even the ones that seem crazy, and challenge our thinking – because UFOs cannot possibly be one thing, but rather a variety of different things, from the mundane to the paranormal. The same rule applies to SP attacks. Some of them could be caused by thought-forms, others by malicious earth-bound spirits, while others may result from a "consciousness split" between our astral and physical bodies, as happened to Monroe on several occasions. Then there's the "right hemispheric intrusion" theory, which, in my opinion, deserves serious scientific study. I feel, however, that the workings of the brain can only tell us so much about SP, and that, should we wish to gain any real understanding of the phenomenon, we must first advance our knowledge of the astral body and the OBE state.

In *Beyond the Occult*, in a chapter that deals with hypnagogic phenomena, Wilson suggests that "deliberately-induced hypnagogia might be the open sesame to the whole field of the paranormal," and that "it could well be the breakthrough that psychic research has been hoping for since the 1880s." Wilson discusses the work of Dr. Andreas Mavromatis of Brunel University, who, having extensively investigated the hypnagogic state by teaching himself and his students how to induce it, discovered that it encourages psi. As detailed in his book *Hypnagogia* (1987), Mavromatis conducted numerous telepathy experiments with his students, whereby the subject – while in a hypnagogic state – attempted to "pick up" various scenes envisaged by the agent. Some of the results were very impressive and could not have been due to coincidence. Mavromatis concluded that "some seemingly 'irrelevant' hypnagogic images might…be meaningful phenomena belonging to another mind."

In *Beyond the Occult*, Wilson mentions how, as observed by Playfair, poltergeist activity tends to occur more frequently when those involved in the haunting are either falling asleep or waking up. This, assumed Playfair, can be explained by the fact that poltergeists generally wish to avoid being observed doing things – and, for example, are more likely to throw objects about when people have their heads turned the other way. Wilson puts forward another theory: "If the twilight state between sleeping and waking makes human beings more 'psychic' (i.e. allows them entry into another condition of being), then it may be a two-way door that also allows the denizens of the psychic realm to invade the physical realm."

Because the SP state is basically a hypnopompic/hypnagogic trance and can sometimes last for an extremely long duration, it could well be not only the most direct and steady portal into the spirit realm – as well as the perfect condition in which to gain information psychically – but, if Wilson's theory has any merit, the main means by which spirits, alien beings, and maybe even UFOs are able to enter and leave our dimension. This isn't much different than the "unconscious medium theory" of poltergeist disturbances. If we're able to "visit" these entities and their world by entering a portal in our minds (what Gooch calls the "inner universe"), perhaps they make use of this very same portal in order to "visit" us. This might explain why, at the beginning of an alien abduction experience as well as at the end, the abductee is usually in a SP-like state. Could it be that abductees are unconscious mediums for these entities? Perhaps, collectively speaking, humanity is a medium for all types of paranormal beings.

Beginning in 1964 and extending over a period of ten years, a series of impressive "dream telepathy" experiments were conducted by Dr. Stanley Krippner and Dr. Montague Ullman at the Maimonides Medical Centre, New York City. The agents – or "senders" – were instructed to influence the dreams of others who were currently asleep (and in an REM state), by transmitting images of art prints, among other things. Later, the subjects – the "receivers" – were roused from sleep and asked to describe what they'd just dreamt about. It was hoped that the transmitted images and such would show up in their dreams – and indeed at times they did. Most of the experiments yielded statistically significant results, indicating that REM sleep is conducive to psi.

It makes senses that the ability of someone in this condition to pick up information telepathically would be far, far greater than that of someone in the typical REM state because the SP state involves a profound degree of awareness during REM sleep. Given the fact that it's possible to trigger SP episodes in SP sufferers, by yanking them out of REM sleep, why not conduct an experiment to see if SP sufferers can read the minds of others? Such an experiment, if done properly, could be extremely successful.

I've thought long and hard about the importance of this book – and indeed the importance of the SP phenomenon – and why I felt the need to write it. And I think I now know. The findings in this book demonstrate that there exists another reality – a "spirit realm" – impinging upon our own, whose inhabitants influence us profoundly and play a much larger role in our lives than we care to imagine – or are able to comprehend. Being an SP sufferer has enabled me to become aware of this reality, not in an abstract sense, but in a factual sense. It has also enabled me to realize that the soul exists and can be understood. As I wrote in the second chapter of this book, during the SP state, you are conscious of the fact that you possess a "soul." Terrifying though my SP experiences have been, I would not have found my soul had they never occurred.

I realize, of course, that many of us – perhaps most of the world's population – believe in some kind of spirit realm or afterlife and also accept the existence of the soul. However, when I say that the SP phenomenon has enabled me to find my soul, I'm doing much more than simply acknowledging my spirituality, or implying that I've had a "spiritual awakening." You could have a "spiritual awakening" as a result of frolicking naked through a field of poppies on a spring morning. I'm using the word "soul" in a very literal sense. As I'm sure many SP sufferers would agree, the SP state puts you in direct contact with your soul, allowing you to experience the spirit realm first-hand. This is immensely significant – even revolutionary.

Acknowledgments

I'd like to thank a number of individuals for helping make this book a reality. They are, in no special order:

My family, especially my sister Kathleen Proud, for identifying a number of errors in the first draft;

Paul McLean, friend and spiritual ally, for the constructive criticism, harsh though it was;

David and Robert from *New Dawn* magazine, especially the former, for believing in my writing and helping me hone my skills. If you hadn't spurred me on, David, much of the material in this book would never have been written. May the *New Dawn* crew – and the magazine itself – live long and prosper!

Colin Wilson, for reading my work and taking it seriously, small fry though I am, and for kindly agreeing to write a foreword;

David J. Hufford, for all the inspiration, for critiquing the book and suggesting ways to improve it, and for kindly agreeing to write the other foreword;

J. Allan Cheyne, for allowing me to quote extensively from his work, namely the University of Waterloo's Sleep Paralysis webpage;

Aeolus Kephas, for generously proving me with an original and fascinating description of his SP experiences;

Patrick Huyghe, for agreeing to publish this crazy book of mine, and for doing such a fine job of it;

All the author/researchers – both dead and alive – whose work I have drawn from, learnt from, and admire, primarily those who have contributed much to our understanding of paranormal and occult phenomena, among them Stan Gooch, Whitley Strieber, Guy Lyon Playfair, Trevor James Constable, Joe Fisher, Wilson Van Dusen, Robert Monroe, Dion Fortune, D. Scott Rogo, Vusamazulu Credo Mutwa, John E. Mack, John A. Keel, Chico Xavier, Allan Kardec, Emmanuel Swedenborg, and anyone else I may have left out by mistake;

Last but not least, Tseada Zekarias, for acquainting me with truth and beauty.

Bibliography

INTERNET:

Paranormal Review, "Enfield Poltergeist Lives Again," March 7, 2007, http://www.paranormalreview.co.uk/News/tabid/59/newsid368/94/Enfield-poltergeist-lives-again/Default.aspx

BBC, h2g2, "Sleep Paralysis," January 2006, http://www.bbc.co.uk/dna/h2g2/A6092471

Tibetan Government in Exile, "Nechung – The State Oracle of Tibet," http://www.tibet.com/Buddhism/nechung_hh.html

SpiritWritings, "Francisco de Paula Candido Xavier," http://www.spiritwritings.com/chicoxavier.html

Adachi, Ken, *Educate-Yourself*, "Trevor James Constable, A Man of Seasons," January 6, 2003, http://educate-yourself.org/tjc/briefbio.shtml

Bellos, Alex, *The Guardian*, "Chico Xavier," July 11, 2002, http://www.guardian.co.uk/news/2002/jul/11/guardianobituaries.booksobituaries1

Blackmore, Susan, Committee for Skeptical Inquiry (CSICOP), "Abduction by Aliens or Sleep Paralysis?" 1998, http://www.csicop.org/si/9805/abduction.html

Blackmore, Susan, "Alien Abduction – The Inside Story," (originally published in *New Scientist*, November 19, 1991), http://www.susanblackmore.co.uk/Articles/alienabduction.html

Blackmore, Susan, "OBEs and Sleep Paralysis," http://www.susanblackmore.co.uk/Conferences/SPR99.html

Blackmore, Susan, *Spiritwatch*, "Lucid Dreams and OBEs," http://sawka.com/spiritwatch/luciddreams.htm

Bower, Bruce, *Science News*, "Night of the Crusher: The Waking

Nightmare of Sleep Paralysis Propels People Into a Spirit World," July 9, 2005, http://findarticles.com/p/articles/mi_m1200/is_2_168/ai_n14863976

Brenner, Keri, *The Olympian*, "Disillusioned Former Students Target Ramtha," 2008, http://www.theolympian.com/570/story/339950.html

Bruce, Robert, *Astral Dynamics*, "Thoughts and Ideas and Frequently Asked Questions," 2004, http://www.astraldynamics.com/tutorials/?BoardID=111

Casteel, Sean, Sean Casteel UFO Journalist, "Whitley Strieber and the Toronto Experience," www.seancasteel.com/toronto.htm

Cheyne, J. Allan, "A Webpage About Sleep Paralysis and Associated Hypnopompic and Hypnagogic Experiences," http://watarts.uwaterloo.ca/~acheyne/S_P.html

Coleman, Loren, *The Anomalist*, "The Sudden Death of Joe Fisher," http://www.anomalist.com/milestones/fisher.html

Davies, Owen, *Folklore*, "The Nightmare Experience, Sleep Paralysis, and Witchcraft Accusations – Focus on 'the Nightmare,'" August 2003, http://findarticles.com/p/articles/mi_m2386

Devali, Allesandra, Brazzil, "Chico of the Spirits," http://www.brazzil.com/p06aug02.htm

Dieckmann, Hans, Answers.com, "Psychoanalysis: Shadow (Analytical Psychology)," http://www.answers.com/topic/shadow

Gillis, Lucy, *The Lucid Dream Exchange*, "Scared Stiff - Sleep Paralysis, An Interview with Jorge Conesa, Ph.D.," 2001, http://www.dreaminglucid.com/articlejc.html

Khamsi, Roxanne, BioEd Online, "Electrical Brainstorms Busted as Source of Ghosts," MacMillan Publishers Ltd., 2004, http://www.bioedonline.org/news/news.cfm?art=1424

Kristof, Nicholas D., *The New York Times*, "Alien Abduction? Science Calls It Sleep Paralysis," July 6, 1999, http://www.nytimes.com/1999/07/06/science/alien-abduction-science-calls-it-sleep-paralysis.html

Lydgate, Chris, *Willamette Week*, "What the #$*! is Ramtha," 2004, http://wweek.com/story.php?story=5860

Moore, Victoria, *Daily Mail*, "The Woman Who Needs a Veil of Protection From Modern Life," April 27, 2007, http://www.dailymail.co.uk/femail/article-450995/The-woman-needs-veil-protection-modern-life.html

Penman, Danny, *Daily Mail*, "Suburban Poltergeist: A 30-year Silence is Broken," March 2007, http://www.dailymail.co.uk/pages/live/articles/news/news.html?in_article_id=440048&in_page_id=1770

Persinger, Dr. M.A., "The Most Frequent Criticisms and Questions Concerning The Tectonic Strain Hypothesis," 1999, http://www.shaktitechnology.com/tectonic.htm

Sherwood, Simon J., "Relationship Between the Hypnagogic/Hypnopompic States and Reports of Anomalous Experiences," http://www.geocities.com/soho/gallery/3549/pa_sp3.html

Strieber, Whitley, *Whitley Strieber's Unknown Country*, "Journey to Another World," March 12, 2004, http://www.unknowncountry.com/journal/?id=149

Suhotra Swami, "Channeling – Extrasensory Deception?" 1998, http://krishnascience.com/Vaisnava%20Library/Philosophy/Articles%20from%20Suhotra%20Swami/Channeling.htm

Swedenborg, Emanuel, *The Heavenly Doctrines*, http://www.heavenlydoctrines.org/

Weinberger, Sharon, *Washington Post*, "Mind Games," January 14, 2007, http://www.washingtonpost.com/wp-dyn/content/article/2007/01/10/AR2007011001399.html

Zap, Jonathan, Zaporacle, *The Siren Call of Hungry Ghosts*, 2006, http://www.zaporacle.com/textpattern/article/110/the-siren-call-of-hungry-ghosts

ARTICLES AND PAPERS

"Sleep Paralysis – Unable to Speak, Unable to Move and All You Did Was Wake Up," *American Academy of Neurology*, April 1, 1999

Bloom, Joseph D. and Gelardin, Richard D., "Eskimo Sleep Paralysis," (date of publication unknown)

Cheyne, J. Allan, "The Ominous Numinous Sensed Presence and 'Other' Hallucinations," *Journal of Consciousness Studies*, 8, No. 5–7, 2001

Hume, Steve, "The Career of 'Allan Kardec,'" *The Ark Review*, Dec. 1997

Jedd, Marcia, "When Ghosts Attack," *Fate*, November 1998

Marcus, Adam, "Ghost Lusters: If You Want to See a Specter Badly Enough, Will You?" *Scientific American*, October 27, 2008

Playfair, Guy Lyon, "The Way of the Spirit," *The Unexplained*, Vol. 3, Issue 26, 1981

Proud, Louis, "The Enfield Poltergeist Revisited," *Fate*, October 2007

Proud, Louis, "Poltergeists," *Fate*, January 2008

Proud, Louis, "Forces of the Unconscious Mind: Exploring the Work of Stan Gooch," *New Dawn*, No. 105, Nov.-Dec. 2007

Proud, Louis, "Haunted by Hungry Ghosts: The Joe Fisher Story," *New Dawn*, Special Issue No. 5, Winter 2008

Proud, Louis, "Allan Kardec and the Way of the Spirit," *New Dawn*, Special Issue No. 5, Winter 2008

Proud, Louis, "Aliens, Predictions & the Secret School: Decoding the Work of Whitley Strieber," *New Dawn*, Special Issue No. 4, Spring 2008

Proud, Louis, "Mind Parasites & the World of Invisible Spirits," *New Dawn*, Special Issue No. 3, Winter 2007

Proud, Louis, "Chico Xavier: The Pope of Spiritism," *New Dawn*, Special Issue No. 6, 2008

Terrillon, Jean-Christophe and Marques-Bonham, Sirley, "Does Recurrent Isolated Sleep Paralysis Involve More Than Cognitive Neurosciences?" *Journal of Scientific Exploration*, Vol. 15, No. 1, 2001

BOOKS:

Penguin English Dictionary, Penguin Books Ltd., UK, 2001

Bruce, Robert, *Astral Dynamics: A New Approach to Out-of-Body Experiences*, Hampton Roads Publishing Company, Inc., USA, 1999

Buhlman, William L., *Adventures Beyond the Body: How to Experience Out-of-Body Travel*, HarperCollins, USA, 1996

Budden, Albert, *UFOs: Psychic Close Encounters*, Blandford, UK, 1995

Budden, Albert, *Electric UFOs: Fireballs, Electromagnetics, and Abnormal States*, Blandford, UK, 1998

Campbell, R.J., *Psychiatric Dictionary*, Oxford University Press, USA, 1996

Catoe, Lynn E., *UFOs and Related Subjects: An Annotated Bibliography*, Gale Group, USA, 1978

Constable, Trevor James, *The Cosmic Pulse of Life: The Revolutionary Biological Power Behind UFOs*, Borderland Sciences Research Foundation, USA, 1976

DeMeo, James, Ph.D., *The Orgone Accumulator Handbook: Construction*

Plans, Experimental Use and Protection Against Toxic Energy, Natural Energy Works, USA, 1989

Fadiman, James, and Kewman, Donald: *Exploring Madness: Experience Theory and Research*, Wadsworth Publishing, California, 1973

Fisher, Joe, *The Siren Call of Hungry Ghosts: A Riveting Investigation Into Channeling and Spirit Guides*, Paraview Press, USA, 2001

Fodor, Nandor, *The Haunted Mind*, Garrett Publications, USA, 1959

Fortune, Dion, *The Mystical Qabalah*, Williams and Norgate, Ltd., UK, 1935

Fortune, Dion, *Psychic Self-Defence: A Study in Occult Pathology and Criminality*, Society of the Inner Light, UK, 1930

Fortune, Dion, *Sane Occultism*, The Society of the Inner Light, UK, 1967

Gardiner, Phillip, and Osborne, Gary, *The Shining Ones: The World's Most Powerful Secret Society Revealed*, Watkins Publishing, UK, 2006

Gooch, Stan, *The Origins of Psychic Phenomena: Poltergeists, Incubi, Succubi, and the Unconscious Mind*, Rider & Co, UK, 1984

Gooch, Stan, *The Paranormal*, Wildwood House, Ltd, 1978

Gyatso, Tenzin (the 14th Dalai Lama), *Freedom in Exile: The Autobiography of the Dalai Lama*, Hodder and Stoughton Ltd., UK, 1990

Harner, Michael, *The Way of the Shaman*, Harper & Row, USA, 1980

Hufford, David J., *The Terror That Comes in the Night: An Experienced-Centered Study of Supernatural Assault Traditions*, University of Pennsylvania Press, USA, 1982

Inglis, Brian, *Trance: A Natural History of Altered States of Mind* (Grafton Books, UK, 1989)

Jaynes, Julian, *The Origin of Consciousness in the Breakdown of the Bicameral Mind*, First Mariner Books, 1976

Kardec, Allan, *The Spirits' Book*, Brotherhood of Life, Inc., USA, 1989

Kardec, Allan, *The Mediums' Book*, Psychic Press Ltd, London, 1971

Keel, John A., *The Mothman Prophecies*, Tom Doherty Associates, LLC, USA, 1975

Klimo, Jon, *Channeling: Investigations On Receiving Information From Paranormal Sources*, Jeremy P. Tarcher, Inc., USA, 1987

Long, Max Freedom, *The Secret Science Behind Miracles: Unveiling the Huna Tradition of the Ancient Polynesians*, DeVorss & Company, USA, 1948

McGregor, Pedro and Smith, T. Stratton, *The Moon and Two Mountains: The Myths, Ritual and Magic of Brazilian Spiritism*, Souvenir Press Ltd., UK, 1966

Mack, John E., *Passport to the Cosmos: Human Transformation and Alien Encounters*, Crown Publishers, USA, 1999

Marrs, Jim, *Alien Agenda*, HarperCollins, USA, 1997

Mavromatis, Andreas, *Hypnagogia*, Routledge & Kegan Paul, London and New York, 1987

Monroe, Robert A., *Journeys Out of the Body*, Doubleday, USA, 1971

Monroe, Robert A., *Far Journeys*, Doubleday, USA, 1985

Monroe, Robert A., *Ultimate Journey*, Doubleday, USA, 1994

Mutwa, Vusamazulu Credo, *Zulu Shaman: Dreams, Prophecies, and Mysteries*, Destiny Books, USA, 1996

Playfair, Guy Lyon, *This House is Haunted: The Investigation Into the*

Enfield Poltergeist, Souvenir Press Ltd., UK, 1980

Playfair, Guy Lyon, *The Flying Cow*, Souvenir Press Ltd., UK, 1975

Playfair, Guy Lyon and Hill, Scott, *The Cycles of Heaven: Cosmic Forces and What They Are Doing to You*, Souvenir Press Ltd., UK, 1978

Pope, Nick, *The Uninvited*, Simon & Schuster, UK, 1997

Randle, Kevin D. and Estes, Russ and Cone, William P., Ph.D., *The Abduction Enigma: The Truth Behind the Mass Alien Abductions of the Late Twentieth Century*, Tom Doherty Associates, LLC, USA, 1999

Regardie, Israel, *The Middle Pillar: The Balance Between Mind and Magic*, Llewellyn Publications, USA, 1970

Rogo, D. Scott, *The Infinite Boundary: Spirit Possession, Madness, and Multiple Personality*, Dodd, Mead & Co, USA, 1987

Rogo, D. Scott, *The Poltergeist Experience: Investigations Into Ghostly Phenomena*, Penguin Books Ltd., UK, 1979

Sevilla, Jorge Conesa, Ph.D., *Wrestling With Ghosts: A Personal and Scientific Account of Sleep Paralysis*, Xlibris Corporation, USA, 2004

Smith, Daniel B., *Muses, Madmen, and Prophets: Rethinking the History, Science, and Meaning of Auditory Hallucinations*, The Penguin Press, USA, 2007

Strieber, Whitley, *Communion: A True Story*, Century, UK, 1987

Strieber, Whitley, *Transformation: The Breakthrough*, Century Hutchinson Ltd., 1988

Strieber, Whitley, *The Secret School: Preparation for Contact*, Simon & Schuster, UK, 1997

Strieber, Whitley, *The Grays*, Tom Doherty Associates, LLC, UK, 2006

Strieber, Whitley, *The Key*, Walker & Collier, Inc., USA, 2001

Synnestvedt, Sig, *The Essential Swedenborg*, Swedenborg Foundation, USA, 1984

Van Dusen, Wilson, *The Natural Depth in Man*, Harper & Row, USA, 1972

Watson, Lyall, *Supernature: A Natural History of the Supernatural*, Hodder and Stoughton Limited, UK, 1973

Wilson, Colin, *The Occult: The Ultimate Book for Those Who Would Walk with the Gods*, Grafton Books, UK, 1979

Wilson, Colin, *Beyond the Occult*, Caxton Editions, London, 1988

Wilson, Colin, *Poltergeist!: A Study in Destructive Haunting*, Claxton Editions, UK, 1981

Wilson, Colin, *Afterlife: An Investigation of the Evidence for Life After Death*, The Leisure Circle Limited, UK, 1985

Wilson, Colin, and Wilson, Damon, The *Mammoth Encyclopedia of Unsolved Mysteries*, Constable and Robinson Ltd., UK, 2000

Xavier, Francisco Candido (by the spirit Andre Luiz), *In The Domain of Mediumship: Life in the Spiritual World*, International Spiritist Council, Brazil, 2006

Xavier, Francisco Candido, (by the spirit Andre Luiz), *The Astral City: The Story of a Doctor's Odyssey in the Spirit World* (originally titled *Nosso Lar*), Spiritist Group of New York and GEAE, 2000, http://www.geae.inf.br/en/books/ac/index.html

CPSIA information can be obtained at www.ICGtesting.com
Printed in the USA
BVOW06s0548200516

448570BV00010B/203/P